Clinical guidelines for chronic conditions in the European Union

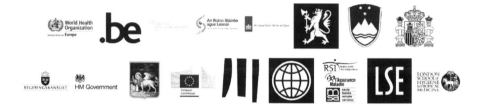

The European Observatory on Health Systems and Policies supports and promotes evidence-based health policy-making through comprehensive and rigorous analysis of health systems in Europe. It brings together a wide range of policy-makers, academics and practitioners to analyse trends in health reform, drawing on experience from across Europe to illuminate policy issues.

The European Observatory on Health Systems and Policies is a partnership, hosted by the World Health Organization Regional Office for Europe, which includes the Governments of Belgium, Finland, Ireland, the Netherlands, Norway, Slovenia, Spain, Sweden, the United Kingdom and the Veneto Region of Italy; the European Commission; the European Investment Bank; the World Bank; UNCAM (French National Union of Health Insurance Funds); the London School of Economics and Political Science; and the London School of Hygiene & Tropical Medicine.

Clinical guidelines for chronic conditions in the European Union

Edited by

**Helena Legido-Quigley, Dimitra Panteli, Josip Car,
Martin McKee, Reinhard Busse**

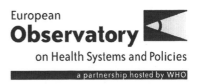

European
Observatory
on Health Systems and Policies
a partnership hosted by WHO

Keywords:
CHRONIC DISEASE – prevention and control
CHRONIC DISEASES AND THEIR CONTROL
DIABETES MELLITUS, TYPE 2
EVIDENCE-BASED MEDICINE
GUIDELINES

This study was commissioned by the European Commission's Directorate-General for Health and Consumers from the European Observatory on Health Systems and Policies as part of a rapid-response (an Observatory mechanism that provides quick evidence reviews to address topical policy questions). It benefited from synergies with the networks and research activities of the ECAB/EUCBCC project on EU Cross Border Care Collaboration (2010–2013), which was co-funded through the EU FP7 Cooperation Work Programme: Health (contract number 242058 and contract acronym EUCBCC).

The European Commission is not responsible for the content of this study, nor for any use of the information it contains. Responsibility for the facts described and the views expressed in it rests entirely with the authors.

ISBN 978 92 890 0021 5

Printed in the United Kingdom

Cover design by M2M

Contents

List of tables, figures and boxes

Boxes

List of abbreviations

ACGBI	Association of Coloproctology of Great Britain and Ireland
ACSS	government contracting department (Portugal)
ADA	American Diabetes Association
ADAPTE	guideline adaptation collaboration
AFSSAPS	French Health Products Safety Agency
AGENAS	National Agency for Regional Healthcare Systems (Italy)
AGREE	Appraisal of Guidelines for Research and Evaluation (instrument)
ALB	arms-length body
ANSM	National Security Agency of Medicines and Health Products (France)
APMGF	Portuguese Association of General and Family Medicine
ARH	Regional Hospital Agencies
ASPP	Austrian Society of Psychiatry and Psychotherapy
AWMF	Association of the Scientific Medical Societies (Germany)
ÄZQ	German Agency for Quality in Medicine
BÄK	German Medical Association
BAPCOC	Belgian Antibiotic Policy Coordination Committee
BIQG	Federal Institute for Quality Assurance in Health Care
BMG	Austrian Federal Ministry of Health
BMI	body mass index
BSG	British Society of Gastroenterology
BTS	British Thoracic Society
CAHIAQ	Catalan Agency for Health Information, Assessment and Quality (former Catalan Agency for Health Technology Assessment, CAHTA)
CBA	controlled before-and-after (trial/study)
CBO	Dutch Institute for Healthcare Improvement (Netherlands)
CCT	controlled clinical trial
CEA	cost–effectiveness analysis
CEBAM	Belgian Centre for Evidence-Based Medicine
CEIPC	Spanish Interdisciplinary Committee for Cardiovascular Disease Prevention
CeVeAs	Centre for the Evaluation of the Effectiveness of Health Care (Italy)
CFS/ME	chronic fatigue syndrome/myalgic encephalomyelitis
CGCC	Clinical Guideline Coordinating Committee (Malta)
CHE	Centre of Health Economics (Latvia) (In November 2011 the Latvian National Health service took over the functions formerly carried out by the Centre of Health Economics)
COPD	chronic obstructive pulmonary disease

CoPFiP	College of Family Physicians (Poland)
CPG	Committee for Practice Guidelines
c-RCT	cluster randomized controlled trial
DACEHTA	Danish Centre for Health Technology Assessment
DDG	German Diabetes Association
DELBI	German Instrument for Methodological Guideline Appraisal
DGS	Directorate-General for Health (Portugal)
DSAM	Danish College of General Practitioners
DVT	deep vein thrombosis
EBMeDS	Evidence-Based Medicine electronic Decision Support system
EBMPracticeNet	Belgian EBM collaboration
EBRO	Dutch national IT platform for clinical guidelines
ECG	electrocardiogram
EHIF	Estonian Health Insurance Fund
ESCARDIO	European Society of Cardiology
ESQH	European Society of Quality in Healthcare
EU	European Union
EULAR	European League Against Rheumatism
FAGP	Flemish Association for General Practice
FBG	fasting blood glucose
FDA	Flemish Diabetes Association
G-BA	Federal Joint Committee (Germany)
GCC	German guideline clearinghouse
GDG	guideline development group
G-I-N	Guidelines International Network
GmbH	Austrian Health Institute
GOAL	platform for guideline implementation (Italy)
GuíaSalud	Clinical Practice Guideline Library for the Spanish National Health System
GYEMSZI	National Institute for Quality and Organizational Development in Healthcare and Medicines (Hungary)
HAS	French National Authority for Health
HDL	high-density lipoprotein
HIQA	Health Information and Quality Authority (Ireland)
HSE	Health Service Executive (Ireland)
HTA	health technology assessment
IAD	Italian Association of Diabetologists
IOM	Institute of Medicine
IPCRG	International Primary Care Respiratory Group
IQWiG	Institute for Quality and Efficiency in Health Care (Germany)
ISD	Italian Society of Diabetology
ISQuA	International Society of Quality in Healthcare
ISS	National Institute of Health (Italy)
IT	information technology
ITS	interrupted time series

JNC	Joint National Committee on Prevention, Detection, Evaluation, and Treatment of High Blood Pressure (United States)
KBV	National Association of Statutory Health Insurance Physicians (Germany)
KCE	Belgian Health Care Knowledge Centre/Federal Centre of Health Care Expertise
KNGF	Royal Dutch Society for Physical Therapy
LEVV	Netherlands Centre for Excellence in Nursing
NABHC	National Advisory Board of Health Care (Hungary)
NBHW	National Board of Health and Welfare
NCC	national collaborating centre
NCCCC	National Collaborating Centre for Chronic Conditions
NCCWCH	National Collaborating Centre for Women's and Children's Health (NICE)
NCD	noncommunicable disease
NCEC	National Clinical Effectiveness Committee (Ireland)
NCEP	National Cholesterol Education Program (National Heart, Lung, and Blood Institute)
NHG	Dutch College of General Practitioners
NHIF	National Health Insurance Fund (Bulgaria)
NHIS	National Health Insurance Scheme (Cyprus)
NHS	National Health Service (Latvia, United Kingdom)
NHS/CKS	National Health Service (United Kingdom) Clinical Knowledge Summaries
NICE	National Institute for Health and Clinical Excellence
NIHDI	National Institute for Health and Disability Insurance (Belgium)
NIKI	National Institute of Quality and Innovations (Slovakia)
NRC	National Reference Centre
NVL	National disease management guidelines (Germany)
OSTEBA	Basque Office for Health Technology Assessment
PCT	Primary Care Trust
PRISMA	Preferred Reporting Items for Systematic Reviews and Meta-Analyses
RCP	Royal College of Physicians
RCT	randomized controlled trial
RIVM	National Institute for Public Health and the Environment (Netherlands)
RR	relative risk
SALAR	Swedish Association of Local Authorities and Regions
SBU	Swedish Council on Health Technology Assessment
SIGN	Scottish Intercollegiate Guidelines Network
SIQuAS-VRQ	Italian Society for Quality in Healthcare
SMPA	Swedish Medical Products Agency
SNLG	National Guideline System (Italy)
THL	National Institute for Health and Welfare
UETS	Health Technology Assessment Unit (Lain Entralgo Agency, Spain)
WONCA	World Organization of National Colleges, Academies and Academic Associations of General Practitioners/Family Physicians

About the editors

Dr Helena Legido-Quigley, London School of Hygiene & Tropical Medicine, London, United Kingdom

Dr Dimitra Panteli, Department of Health Care Management, Berlin University of Technology, Berlin, Germany

Dr Josip Car, Global eHealth Unit, Imperial College London, and Imperial College Healthcare NHS Trust, London, United Kingdom

Professor Martin McKee, London School of Hygiene & Tropical Medicine, and European Observatory on Health Systems and Policies, London, United Kingdom

Professor Reinhard Busse, European Observatory on Health Systems and Policies, and Berlin University of Technology, Berlin, Germany

About the chapter authors

Dr Helena Legido-Quigley, London School of Hygiene & Tropical Medicine, London, United Kingdom

Dr Dimitra Panteli, Department of Health Care Management, Berlin University of Technology, Berlin, Germany

Dr Serena Brusamento, Imperial College London, London, United Kingdom

Dr Cécile Knai, London School of Hygiene & Tropical Medicine, London, United Kingdom

Dr Vanessa Saliba, London School of Hygiene & Tropical Medicine, London, United Kingdom

Ms Meritxell Solé, University of Barcelona, Barcelona, Spain

Ms Eva Turk, DNV Research and Innovation, Healthcare programme, Oslo, Norway

Ms Uta Augustin, Department of Health Care Management, Berlin University of Technology, Berlin, Germany

Dr Josip Car, Global eHealth Unit, Imperial College London, and Imperial College Healthcare NHS Trust, London, United Kingdom

Professor Martin McKee, London School of Hygiene & Tropical Medicine, and European Observatory on Health Systems and Policies, London, United Kingdom

Professor Reinhard Busse, European Observatory on Health Systems and Policies, and Berlin University of Technology, Berlin, Germany

International contributors

Dr Luisa Pettigrew, General practitioner, NHS, United Kingdom

Dr Charilaos Lygidakis, General practitioner, Regional Health Service of Emilia-Romagna, Italy

Ms Ilaria Passarani, The European Consumers' Organisation (BEUC), Brussels, Belgium

Mr Willy Palm, European Observatory on Health Systems and Policies, and WHO European Centre for Health Policy, Brussels, Belgium

About the country profile authors

Austria

Ms Andrea Schmidt, Health and Care Department European Centre for Social Welfare Policy and Research, Vienna

Dr Christian Claus Schiller, General practitioner, Bad Schallerbach Department of Medicine, General Hospital of the Barmherzige Schwestern, Linz

Dr Georg Ruppe, Health and Care Department European Centre for Social Welfare Policy and Research, Vienna

Belgium

Dr Aldo Perissino, Acute, Chronic and Elderly Care Policy Unit, DG Organisation of Healthcare Establishments, FPS Health, Food Chain Safety and Environment, Brussels

Mr Miguel Lardennois, Acute, Chronic and Elderly Care Policy Unit, DG Organisation of Healthcare Establishments, FPS Health, Food Chain Safety and Environment, Brussels

Dr Carls Steylaerts, MD, Diest

Professor Dr Paul Van Royen, Department of Primary and Interdisciplinary Care, University of Antwerp, Antwerp

Ms Muriel Quinet, DG Primary Health Care Services and Crisis Management, Strategic Coordination of Health Professionals, FPS Health, Food Chain Safety and Environment, Brussels

Dr Margareta Haelterman, Acute Chronic and Elderly Care Policy Unit, DG Organisation of Healthcare Establishments, FPS Health, Food Chain Safety and Environment, Brussels

Dr Pascal Meeus, Health Services Department, Direction Research, Development and Quality, National Institute for Health and Disability Insurance, Brussels

Bulgaria

Professor Antoniya Dimova, Department of Health Economics and Management, Varna University of Medicine, Varna

Cyprus

Mr Mamas Theodorou, Open University of Cyprus, Latsia

Czech Republic

Dr Ales Bourek, Masaryk University, Brno

Denmark

Mr Steen Dalsgård Jespersen, Primary and Community Health Care, National Board of Health, Copenhagen

Dr Jette Blands, Department of Environmental and Structural Health, National Board of Health, Copenhagen

Estonia

Mr Jarno Habicht, WHO Country Office for Estonia, Tallinn

Dr Ain Aaviksoo, PRAXIS Centre for Policy Studies, Tallinn

Finland

Dr Anna-Mari Aalto, Service System Research Unit, National Institute Health and Welfare, Helsinki

Dr Jorma Komulainen, Finnish Medical Society Duodecim, Current Care Guidelines, Helsinki

Dr Suvi Vainiomäki, Department of Health Care and Social Services, Turku

France

Ms Isabelle Clerc-Urmès, Institut National de la Santé et de la Recherche Médicale, Paris

Dr Michel Laurence, Haute Autorité de Santé, Paris

Dr Matthias Brunn, URC Économie de la santé, Université Paris-Est/AP-HP, Paris

Germany

Dr Tobias Freund, Department of General Practice and Health Services Research, University Hospital Heidelberg, Heidelberg

Professor Dr Günter Ollenschläger, Agency for Quality in Medicine (ÄZQ), Berlin

Greece

Dr Athanasios Nikolentzos, Health Services Research, Hellenic Open University, Patras

Dr Kostas Voliotis, Alexandroupolis General Hospital, Alexandroupolis

Hungary

Ms Eszter Kovács, Health Services Management Training Centre, Semmelweis University, Budapest

Ms Blanka Török, Health Services Management Training Centre, Semmelweis University, Budapest

Dr Gábor Szócska MD, Health Services Management Training Centre, Semmelweis University, Budapest

Ireland

Mr Ian Callanan, Clinical Audit, Health Service Executive, St Vincent's Healthcare Group, Dublin

Italy

Professor Piera Poletti, Centro Ricerca e Formazione (CEREF), Padova

Dr Sara Rigon, Regional Health Service of Emilia-Romagna, Bologna

Dr Silva Mitro, Local Health Authority No.10, Veneto Region, San Donà di Piave

Latvia

Ms Inese Arzova, Division of Treatment Quality, Health Care Department of the Ministry of Health, Riga

Ms Antra Valdmane, Division of Treatment Quality, Health Care Department of the Ministry of Health, Riga

Lithuania

Ms Marina Karanikolos, European Observatory on Health Systems and Policies, Research Fellow, London School of Hygiene & Tropical Medicine, United Kingdom

Luxembourg

Dr Martin Sattler, General practitioner, City of Luxembourg

Dr Siggy Rausch, General practitioner, City of Luxembourg

Dr Yolande Wagener, Ministry of Health, City of Luxembourg

Malta

Dr Vanessa Saliba, London School of Hygiene & Tropical Medicine, London, United Kingdom

Dr Natasha Azzopardi Muscat, Strategy and Sustainability Division, Ministry of Health, the Elderly and Community Care, Valletta

Professor Stephen Fava, Diabetes & Endocrine Centre, Mater Dei Hospital, Msida

Dr Gunther Abela, Department of Primary Health, Floriana

Dr Tonio Piscopo, Department of Medicine, Mater Dei Hospital, Msida

Professor Joe Azzopardi, Diabetes & Endocrine Centre, Mater Dei Hospital, Msida

Netherlands

Dr Sietse Wieringa, General practitioner, NHS, London, United Kingdom

Professor Hans Maarse, Faculty of Health Sciences, University of Maastricht, Maastricht

Norway

Dr Robert Anders Burman, National Centre for Emergency Primary Health Care, Bergen

Ms Eva Turk, DNV Research and Innovation, Healthcare programme, Oslo

Poland

Ms Basia Kutryba, National Center for Quality Assessment in Healthcare, Krakow

Ms Halina Wasikowska, National Center for Quality Assessment in Healthcare, Krakow

Mr Piotr Gajewski, *Medycyna Praktyczna [Practical Medicine]*, Krakow

Mr Marek Oleszczyk, Department of Family Medicine, Jagiellonian University, Krakow

Portugal

Dr Tiago Villanueva, General practitioner, Lisbon

Professor Jaime Correia de Sousa, Department of Community Health, School of Health Sciences, Minho University, Braga

Romania

Dr Ionela Petrea, Department of International Development Mental Health, Trimbos Institute, Netherlands Institute for Mental Health and Addiction, Utrecht, Netherlands

Dr Constantinescu Vasilica, National School of Public Health Management and Professional Development, Bucharest

Ms Raluca Sfetcu, National School of Public Health Management and Professional Development, Bucharest

Dr Silvia Forescu, MD, National School of Public Health Management and Professional Development, Bucharest

Slovakia

Ms Henrieta Mádarová, Advance Healthcare Management Institute, Prague, Czech Republic

Dr Lenka Bachrata, General practitioner, Bratislava

Dr Martin Višňanský, General practitioner, Bratislava

Slovenia

Dr Jelka Zaletel, University Clinical Centre, Ljubljana

Spain

Dr Maria-Dolors Estrada, Catalan Agency for Health Information, Assessment and Quality (CAHIAQ), Generalitat of Catalonia Health Department, Barcelona, and GuíaSalud Scientific Committee

Ms Arritxu Etxeberria, Basque Health Service, Gipuzkoa, Basque Country, Health Technology Assessment Unit (UETS), Lain Entralgo Agency, Madrid, and GuíaSalud Scientific Committee

Dr Laura Otero, National School of Public Health, Carlos III Health Institute Instituto de Salud Carlos III, Ministry of Science and Innovation, Madrid

Ms Rosa Rico, Basque Health Technology Assessment Agency, Basque Office for Health Technology Assessment (OSTEBA), Basque Country, Vitoria-Gasteiz, and GuíaSalud Scientific Committee

Ms Meritxell Sole, University of Barcelona, Barcelona

Sweden

Mr Michael Bergstrom, Division of Health and Social Care, Swedish Association of Local Authorities and Regions (SALAR), Stockholm

Dr Lidia Amini, General practitioner, Uppsala

Switzerland

Dr François Héritier, Swiss Association of General Practitioners, Bern

Professor Bernard Burnand, Department of Biology and Medicine, University of Lausanne, Lausanne

United Kingdom (England)

Dr Paula Malongane, General practitioner, NHS, London

Dr Vanessa Saliba, London School of Hygiene & Tropical Medicine, London

Dr Françoise Cluzeau, NICE International, London

Foreword

In Europe today, chronic diseases are the leading cause of illness and disability. Over 100 million citizens or 40% of the population in Europe over the age of 15 are reported to have a chronic disease and two out of three people reaching retirement age will have had at least two chronic conditions.

These diseases by their nature are not easily cured and require long-term medical care. As a result, patients and their families need to adapt their lives in order to manage the disease. This also puts an increasing strain on health systems to cater for these needs. It is widely acknowledged that **70–80% of health care costs are spent on chronic diseases**. This corresponds to €700 billion in the European Union and this number is expected to rise in the coming years.

The role of chronic disease management, including the role of the patient in managing their care, merits more attention. However, we should not allow our continuing focus on prevention to diminish. Despite decades of work in the areas of health promotion and disease prevention, we still have a long way to go in identifying cost-effective actions to address the main risk factors responsible for chronic diseases.

In order to be able to analyse the above-mentioned issues, identify gaps and explore where the European Union's actions should be targeted, the European Commission and the Member States launched a reflection process on chronic diseases. This process, following Council Conclusions in 2010, seeks to explore and disseminate innovative approaches to addressing chronic diseases. It aims to review and galvanize interest in promotion and disease management.

The Commission aims to build on the existing work. For this reason, the Commission requested the European Observatory on Health Systems and Policies to prepare an overview or a compilation of the existing guidelines, which Member States currently have in place to tackle and manage chronic diseases.

I warmly welcome this report prepared by the European Observatory on Health Systems and Policies. The report makes a contribution to our continuing reflection process on chronic diseases by helping us to better understand the European landscape and share stories of success. It illustrates the need for, and the way in which, clinical guidelines can contribute to optimizing processes and to providing higher quality, more effective and more cost-efficient care for patients.

P Testori Coggi, Director-General, Directorate-General for Health and Consumers, European Commission

Executive summary

Introduction

Ageing populations and advances in the scope of medical care combine to create a situation in which chronic noncommunicable diseases are increasingly impacting on European health systems. Chronic noncommunicable diseases require a long-term perspective, not only in tackling their determinants and thus preventing them from occurring, but also in developing the often complex programmes needed to manage them, in which multidisciplinary teams intervene both simultaneously and consecutively. This necessitates a systematic and integrated approach. However, the way that different health systems engage in these efforts and where they place their priorities differs markedly. The European Union – in its role of encouraging exchange of information in support of public health – seeks to facilitate concerted action to optimize responses to the challenges of chronic noncommunicable diseases. This includes identifying innovative methods for cost-effective prevention of common risk factors, for developing coordinated patient-centred care, and for stimulating integrated research. A first step is to gather knowledge on how clinical guidelines for chronic noncommunicable disease prevention and treatment have been developed and implemented in different countries. To this end, the European Commission's Directorate-General for Health and Consumers asked the European Observatory on Health Systems and Policies to prepare a report exploring the various national practices relating to clinical guidelines along with their impact on processes of care and patients' outcomes.

Objectives of the report

This report seeks to understand the definitions used for clinical guidelines relevant to chronic noncommunicable diseases and their relationship with related strategies to improve care for chronically ill patients; the regulatory basis for, actors involved and processes used in developing clinical guidelines across the European Union and the quality thereof; the strategies used to disseminate and implement clinical guidelines in various countries and what is known about their effectiveness; and whether clinical guidelines actually have an impact on processes of care and patients' health outcomes.

Structure of the report

- **Introduction.** The report opens with a brief explanation of the emergence of clinical guidelines in Europe and the evolution of aims and definitions of clinical guidelines over time, placing clinical guidelines within the context of other instruments designed to link research and clinical practice.

- **Mapping exercise and case studies.** The report then describes (i) a summary of clinical guidelines experience in all European countries; and (ii) a more in-depth analysis of the development and use of type 2 diabetes mellitus guidelines in France, Germany, Malta, Slovenia, Spain and the United Kingdom (England). This analysis is conducted according to an agreed conceptual framework designed to assess systematically existing clinical guidelines in the European Union. The conceptual framework consists of six dimensions: background information, regulatory basis, development, quality control, implementation and evaluation of clinical guidelines.

- **Systematic literature review.** The report subsequently presents a systematic literature review of studies analysing (i) the development quality, (ii) the implementation and (iii) the impact of European clinical guidelines for coronary heart disease, chronic obstructive pulmonary disease, asthma, type 2 diabetes mellitus, osteoarthritis, various cancers (breast, cervical and colorectal) and depressive disorder.

- **Conclusions and policy recommendations.** Based on the evidence assembled, the report concludes by summarizing the main findings and proposes policy recommendations at national and European levels, which could improve how clinical guidelines are developed and implemented.

Summary of findings

Mapping exercise and case studies

The mapping exercise provides a thorough and updated account of how clinical guidelines operate in Europe. It illustrates the divergent status of clinical guideline production in the European Union.

- **Range of practice.** The analysis of country responses distinguishes three broad categories of Member State engagement in clinical guideline development. The first category includes those with a long tradition in guideline production and implementation, whereby relevant activities are an established aspect of service provision. The second encompasses those that have started producing and using clinical guidelines but for a more limited range of settings and conditions; and the third category comprises those countries in which only initial steps towards guideline utilization can be identified and those in which initiatives in this area seem to be still in the planning stage.

- **Regulatory framework.** The value of a legal mandate for clinical guideline use is inconclusive: certain countries have relevant laws but those laws may or may not be implemented and, conversely, highly developed systems often function without any legal basis.

- **Bodies responsible for guideline production.** Guidelines are usually developed by government or quasi-governmental organizations and professional associations, often working together. Countries without a comprehensive suite of clinical guidelines, individuals and organizations take guidance from elsewhere, either from pan-European, American bodies or from other countries. Some institutions, besides having their own clinical guideline programmes, also engage internationally with networks established for the purpose of knowledge exchange, methodological development and coordination of care.

- **Stakeholders.** The engagement of stakeholders is a key feature in those few countries with well-established clinical guideline systems, considered to be important to ensure transparency. Depending on the context stakeholders can include representatives of professional organizations, service providers, the pharmaceutical industry and funding bodies; patients, their families and carers and patient representatives or organizations; academics or other experts; and other members of civil society. Their involvement in guidance production varies. In some countries stakeholders are encouraged to use their networks and influence to assist implementation of the clinical guidelines at both national and local levels. In general, patient and service user organizations appear to have little influence in terms of driving the development of clinical guidelines.

- **Quality control and evaluation.** Those few organizations seeking to ascertain the quality of their guidelines often use the well-accepted Appraisal of Guidelines for Research and Evaluation tool, in some cases adapted to context, while others have developed their own approaches. Although some countries have made explicit efforts to appraise clinical guidelines, most countries do not have any formal way to regularly evaluate the development, quality control, implementation and the use of them.

A limitation of this exercise is that while it was possible to collect information about all countries, this information is very general and it does not allow the important practical aspects of the clinical guidelines' "life-cycle" to be ascertained, such as the barriers to implementation, their impact and whether those guidelines that are being developed are of good quality and regularly updated.

Systematic literature review

- **Methodological quality of guidelines.** Four studies analysed the methodological quality of 21 European clinical guidelines focusing on chronic diseases, using the Appraisal of Guidelines for Research and Evaluation tool. The findings confirmed conclusions of other studies; namely, that there was considerable variation in quality. This indicates a lack of consistency in terms of some aspects of the information provided to clinicians across Europe. Inconsistencies in the quality of guidelines may have an impact on the quality of recommendations made and therefore on quality of care provided to patients. Moreover, the findings consistently showed that the least well-addressed domains within the Appraisal of Guidelines for Research and Evaluation tool were stakeholder involvement, rigour of development, applicability and editorial independence.

- **Implementation and impact of guidelines.** Overall only two studies found that the implementation or impact of guidelines was "mostly effective", five studies showed "partial effectiveness" and three studies did not demonstrate any effectiveness. However, the results and the effect size varied across the included studies. The evaluation of the different implementation strategies showed that multifaceted implementation strategies are slightly more effective than single interventions, and continuous feedback and outreach meetings seem to be promising strategies. Included studies did not provide data on the costs relating to the dissemination or implementation of the guidelines. Although resources are essential to generate guidelines, data on the cost of guidelines' development are scarce.

Policy recommendations and research priorities

- **Policy recommendations.** The divergent practices regarding the development, dissemination and implementation of clinical guidelines reflect the different stages of development of quality assurance mechanisms in European health systems. A similar initiative to the one promoting the optimization of health technology assessment methodology (the European Network for Health Technology Assessment programme) for clinical guidelines development would greatly benefit those countries whose guideline development and application are still in their infancy and would support the establishment or amelioration of quality assurance practices.

- **Research priorities.** The mapping exercise within this report highlights a severe lack of evaluated information on what really happens in the majority of countries in Europe. The literature review is especially revealing, illustrating that only a few rigorous studies exist assessing the quality and effectiveness of clinical guidelines in Europe. Further research is needed to support the standardization of guideline terminology; to develop more rigorous studies to evaluate health outcomes associated with the use of clinical guidelines; to assess the cost–effectiveness of guidelines; to investigate the perspective of service users and health service staff; and to conduct more studies evaluating guidelines on prevention, depressive disorder and other mental health conditions.

Part 1

Overview, conceptual framework and methods

H Legido-Quigley, C Knai, D Panteli, M McKee and R Busse

Ageing populations and advances in the scope of medical care combine to create a situation in which chronic noncommunicable diseases (NCDs) are increasingly affecting European health systems. The NCDs examined in this rapid response report are coronary heart disease, chronic obstructive pulmonary disease (COPD), asthma, type 2 diabetes mellitus, osteoarthritis, breast cancer, cervical cancer, colorectal cancer and depressive disorder.

Chronic NCDs require a long-term perspective, first in tackling their determinants and thus preventing them from occurring, but also in developing the often complex programmes needed to manage them, in which different health professionals intervene both simultaneously and consecutively. This necessitates a systematic and integrated approach. However, the way that different health systems engage in these efforts and where they place their priorities differ markedly. The European Union (EU), in its role of exchange of information in support of public health, seeks to facilitate concerted action to optimize responses to the challenges of chronic NCDs. This includes identifying innovative methods for cost-effective prevention of common risk factors, for developing coordinated patient-centred care, and for stimulating integrated research. The first step would be gathering knowledge on how clinical guidelines for chronic NCD prevention and treatment have been developed and implemented in different countries. To this end, the European Commission's Directorate-General for Health and Consumers has asked the European Observatory on Health Systems and Policies to prepare a report exploring the various national practices relating to clinical guidelines, along with their impact on processes of care and patients' outcomes.

This report seeks to understand:

- the definitions used for clinical guidelines relevant to chronic NCDs and their relationship with related strategies to improve care for chronically ill patients;

- the regulatory basis for, actors involved and processes used in developing clinical guidelines across the EU and the quality thereof;

- the strategies used to disseminate and implement clinical guidelines in various countries and what is known about their effectiveness;

- whether clinical guidelines actually have an impact on processes of care and patients' health outcomes.

To do so, the report is organized in the following way. It opens with a brief explanation of the emergence of clinical guidelines in Europe and the evolution of aims and definitions of clinical guidelines over time, situating them within the context of other instruments designed to link research and clinical practice.

The report then describes (i) a summary of clinical guidelines experience in all European countries; and (ii) a more in-depth analysis of the development and use of type 2 diabetes mellitus guidelines in England, France, Germany, Malta, Slovenia and Spain. This analysis is conducted according to a conceptual framework designed to assess systematically existing clinical guidelines in the EU. The conceptual framework consists of six dimensions: background information, regulatory basis, development, quality control, implementation and evaluation of clinical guidelines.

The report subsequently presents a systematic literature review of studies analysing (i) the development quality, (ii) the implementation and (iii) the impact on European clinical guidelines for coronary heart disease, COPD, asthma, type 2 diabetes mellitus, osteoarthritis, various cancers (breast, cervical, and colorectal), and depressive disorder.

Based on the evidence compiled in this report, conclusions are drawn by summarizing the main findings and proposing policy recommendations at both national and European levels, which could improve how clinical guidelines are developed and implemented.

Clinical guidelines: background and overview

This introductory section provides an overview of the historical evolution of clinical guidelines, their aims and conceptualization, along with the way in which they have been appraised and evaluated, while the subsequent section presents the conceptual framework of this report, addressing the issues discussed in this section. Therefore, the aim of this part of the report is to navigate the reader in terms of the evolution of aims and definitions of clinical guidelines over time, placing clinical guidelines within the context of other tools designed to link research and clinical practice.

Evidence-based medicine and clinical guidelines

Clinical guidelines are one of the many tools available to health care professionals, among others, to improve the quality of health care. The Institute of Medicine (IOM) has defined clinical guidelines as "systematically developed statements to assist practitioner and patient decisions about appropriate health care for specific clinical circumstances" (Lohr, 1990). As the IOM definition suggests, clinical guidelines are intended to assist the decision-making process.

Clinical guidelines are derived from the concept of evidence-based medicine. Among the most widely quoted definitions of evidence-based medicine is: "Evidence-based medicine is the conscientious, explicit and judicious use of current best evidence in making decisions about the care of individual patients" (Sackett et al., 1996). In practice, however, this narrow focus is often extended to encompass clinical guidelines directed at groups of patients with a common condition and health technology assessment (HTA), where the focus is on technologies. All these components of evidence-based medicine are committed to improving health through rigorous scientific appraisal (Gupta, 2011).

The emergence of evidence-based medicine in the 1990s (Guyatt, 1991; Guyatt et al., 1992) ushered in an explicit shift towards methodologically critical appraisal of evidence and, specifically, the employment of systematic reviews of relevant literature as the basis for developing valid clinical guidelines (Burgers, Grol et al., 2003b). Evidence-based medicine signifies a shift in decision-making, moving from a reliance on individual clinical expertise towards an application of empirical "collective" evidence to validate clinical decisions (Degen, Hodgins & Bhandari, 2008). In practice, it aims to combine the application of best available scientific evidence, clinical experience and a consideration of patients' values, preferences and expectations (Mayer, 2006) – rather than a cookbook approach (Sackett et al., 1996).

Many factors converged to drive the evidence-based medicine movement, especially the wide variation in medical practice for similar patients (in the literature termed "small-area variation" (Wennberg & Gittelsohn, 1973)), "the harsh reality of medicine ... that many, if not most, daily clinical decisions are not based on valid scientific fact" (McDonald, 1996), an acknowledgement of upward pressure on health care costs – pressure to make the best use of limited resources (value for money) – and a public more engaged in treatment options (McQueen, 2001).

The challenge of ensuring that all medical practice would be based on scientific evidence has been substantial – not least because of the rapidly increasing volume of scientific research and the acknowledgement that many scientific studies are methodologically inadequate, with significant risks of bias and thus potentially misleading. It was thus necessary to form networks and to develop robust methods to assess the quality of studies, and to combine their results in systematic reviews and meta-analyses that would address these challenges. A critical driver for this development was the formation of the Cochrane Collaboration (The Cochrane Collaboration, 2012).

The goal of making the best clinical decision for a patient requires that certain steps are taken. Clinical guidelines contribute to this goal, insofar as their objective is to arrive at an agreement on how patients should be treated (McQueen, 2001). "Evidence" in the context of evidence-based medicine should include evidence not only from the perspective of health care professionals but also patients, taking into account their particular needs, preferences and circumstances (Gupta, 2011; Hewitt-Taylor, 2006). These ethical goals of patient involvement and engagement in their health care are increasingly reflected in the debate on the quality of clinical guidelines; however, consideration of patients' needs and their participation in drawing up clinical guidelines are not yet comprehensively addressed (Gupta, 2011).

The integration of evidence-based medicine with patient needs and treatment preferences depends on informed, engaged patients making decisions at the point of care and at the level of clinical guideline development (Hasnain-Wynia, 2006). A 1998 paper on evidence-based medicine and clinical guidelines notes that, as guidelines were rarely tested in patient care settings prior to publication (as a drug would be before being approved), the quality of clinical guidelines is defined narrowly by an analysis of how closely recommendations are linked to scientific and clinical evidence (Heffner, 1998). This concern remains, although it is now more explicitly addressed, raising the question of whether guidelines should be systematically pilot tested in patient care settings before being approved.

Aims and definitions of clinical guidelines

Clinical guidelines may address various aspects of clinical practice. They can offer instructions on which diagnostic or screening tests need to be ordered, how to provide medical or surgical services, how long patients should stay in hospital, or other details of clinical practice (HIQA, 2011). Clinical guidelines aim to improve the quality of health care and reduce inappropriate variation in health care practice. They can be used to:

- provide recommendations for the treatment and care of people by health professionals

- develop standards to assess the clinical practice of individual health professionals

- help educate and train health professionals

- help patients make informed decisions.

In practice, however, there often seems to be confusion about what the actual meaning of the term is and how it differs from other tools designed to improve the quality of health care. To clarify these issues it is important to examine the most commonly used definitions of the term "clinical guidelines" and compare them with definitions of other terms that have been used interchangeably with them. Table 1.1 provides an overview of the most frequently applied definitions of clinical guidelines as identified in the pertinent literature.

Table 1.1 *Definitions of clinical guidelines*

Author/ Organization	Definition
IOM[a]	Clinical guidelines are systematically developed statements to assist practitioner and patient decisions about appropriate health care for specific clinical circumstances.
SIGN	Clinical guidelines are neither cookbook nor textbook, but where there is evidence of variation in practice which affects patient outcomes and a strong research base providing evidence of effective practice – guidelines can assist health care professionals in making decisions about appropriate and effective care for their patients.
The Canadian Partnership Against Cancer	A set of recommendations about the most appropriate practice for a particular health condition, together with a summary of the evidence that supports the recommendations and a transparent description of the process used to develop them, including how the evidence was interpreted and summarized.
NICE	The NICE's clinical guidelines are recommendations, based on the best available evidence, for the care of people by health care professionals. They are relevant to clinicians, health service managers and commissioners, as well as to patients and their families and carers.
CBO	Guidelines are not laws, but constitute evidence-based statements and recommendations. The recommendations are usually based on the "standard patient" and on the best available evidence. In individual cases, health care professionals could deviate from guideline recommendations based on their professional experience and autonomy.

[a] Field & Lohr, 1990.

The aforementioned definition proposed by the IOM has been particularly influential. Its wording highlights the importance of developing clinical guidelines in a systematic way and it emphasizes how they should be "assisting" and not replacing clinical decisions and those made by patients. The remaining definitions, although with minor differences in wording, also emphasize the idea that clinical guidelines are intended as an aid to clinical judgement, not as a replacement. Furthermore, clinical guidelines should also be of relevance to other stakeholders, including patients and their families and carers (NICE, 2009b). The definition chosen by the Canadian Partnership Against Cancer adds the importance of evidence, clearly stating that the process of clinical guideline development should be carried out in a transparent way (Harrison & Van den Hoek, 2010).

The term "guidelines" implies that their use is voluntary. However, in practice, there is a wide spectrum, ranging from purely voluntary to mandatory (although in the latter case, clinical guidelines should be more precisely termed "directives") and also from the two "anchors" of their development, namely, whether they are based on evidence or consensus (Table 1.2). These differences are sometimes reflected in the different terms used. For example, clinical guidelines used in Belgium can be distinguished as follows: (i) informal consensus-based guidelines, developed by a group of experts based on their opinion and practical experience (closest to field A in the table); (ii) formal consensus-based guidelines, developed using systematic methods to translate expert opinions into recommendations (field E); (iii) evidence-based practice guidelines, developed by a team of clinical and methodological experts, taking into account findings from a systematic literature review, practical experience, values, preferences and circumstances (field H). Some specific directives are called "protocols" and are mandatory; these may be designed by health facilities (for example hospitals) or by health authorities, in which case they are mandatory for every medical institute in the region (as resembled by fields C, F and J in Table 1.2). In Germany, the Association of the Scientific Medical Societies (*Arbeitsgemeinschaft der Wissenschaftlichen Medizinischen Fachgesellschaften*, AWMF) – the umbrella organization of 158 medical societies which coordinates the development of voluntary clinical guidelines on behalf of the medical associations in Germany since 1995 – classifies clinical guidelines as "S2k" if they are based on consensus only (field A); as "S2e" if they are based on best available evidence only (field H in the table) and as "S3" (field D) if both conditions are fulfilled ("S1" is used for expert opinion-based clinical guidelines). Another type of guidelines, the national disease management guidelines (*Nationale Versorgungsleitlinien*, NVL), are developed alongside the Disease Management Programmes (field E) (for further clarification, see the section on Germany in Part 3 of this report). The latter underlines how clinical guidelines may not be explicitly termed as such if they are part of a "package" addressing chronic diseases (for example, Disease Management Programmes or national frameworks within the English National Health Service (NHS)) (NHS Choices, 2012). Typically, their use is then incentivized through the payment system or included as a contractual obligation (fields B, E and I in Table 1.2). If their use is mandatory, they are normally termed "directives".

Table 1.2 *Spectrum of clinical guidelines along the two dimensions "consensus to evidence-based" and "voluntary to mandatory"*

	Purely voluntary	Included in contracts, either incentivized or as an obligatory component	Mandatory by regulation within certain institutions and/ or jurisdictions	Mandatory by law
Purely consensus-based (among potential clinical guideline users)	A	B	C	–
Consensus-based (based upon best available evidence)	D	E	F	G
Purely evidence-based (developed by experts)	H	I	J	K

Another perspective on clinical guidelines is their role in "translation" (Fig. 1.1). Clinical guidelines – together with HTA – form a crucial link between research and practice. Sometimes these terms are confusing because these activities have a common basis in evidence-based medicine, both relying on systematic reviews and meta-analyses of the available evidence to assess the effectiveness and cost–effectiveness of interventions. However, HTA focuses on a particular technology or a group of technologies (for example, drugs, surgical procedures, medical devices) and mainly addresses decision-makers' needs and questions (such as whether to include a technology in the public benefits basket or whether to invest in a certain technology), while clinical guidelines focus on patients' conditions or diseases throughout the entire period of care and primarily address clinicians and patients.

Clinical pathways are related to clinical guidelines and are also referred to as (clinical) protocols, care pathways, integrated pathways, among many synonyms (De Bleser et al., 2006). They tend to focus on the care of patients within one provider institution, with "standards" setting minimum requirements for a provider. Clinical pathways aim to facilitate the introduction of clinical guidelines into clinical practice, and are designed to provide a link between the establishment of clinical guidelines and their use. Moreover, they support communication with and engagement of patients by providing a clearly written summary of their expected care plan and progress over time (Campbell et al.,

1998). In addition, the term "pathways" is also used differently across Europe. For example, in the United Kingdom the term is used to define the graphic descriptions or "algorithms" for both clinical guidelines and clinical pathways.

Fig. 1.1 *The translational pipeline*

From gene discovery to health application		From health application to evidence-based guideline		From guideline to health practice		From practice to health impact
Analytical validation	Clinical utility	Meta-analysis	HTA	Dissemination research	Diffusion research	Outcomes research
Clinical validation	Clinical studies	Systematic reviews	Guideline development	Implementation research		
Human genome epidemiology		Public health genomics		System/ organisation research	Health admin Policy research	Public health genomics

Ethical, legal and social issues

Dissemination of Knowledge research

Source: Adapted from ESF, 2012.

Fig. 1.1 also shows that for clinical guidelines to have a real impact on patient outcomes, it is not enough for them to be developed appropriately; they must also be disseminated and implemented in ways that ensure that they are actually used by clinicians (marked by the dotted area). These issues are addressed in greater detail in the following subsections.

The need to evaluate clinical guidelines

Although evidence-based medicine has contributed to improving the scientific quality of clinical guidelines, the variability of their quality has been a well-documented matter of concern (McGlynn, Kosecoff & Brook, 1990; Audet, Greenfield & Field, 1990) and methodological shortcomings remain a challenge (Heffner, 1998) – a conclusion confirmed by this report. These goals have been reflected in the debate on the quality of clinical guidelines (Gupta, 2011).

Initially, the process of developing clinical guidelines was considered especially important because of the influence this will have on the quality of the evidence that is used and on its effective translation into clinical practice (McQueen, 2001; Shekelle et al., 1999). This is founded on the premise that the greater the strength of the incorporated evidence, the greater the quality of the guideline (McQueen, 2001), and the greater the potential of clinical guidelines to improve the use of resources and quality of health care (Boluyt, Lincke & Offringa, 2005; Woolf et al., 1999; Delgado-Noguera et al., 2009).

Thus far, much work has been carried out to identify the attributes of high-quality clinical guidelines, prompting debate on which quality criteria are most important. Ward & Grieco (1996) proposed applicability, validity (including assessment of strength of evidence), reproducibility, clinical flexibility, clarity, multi-disciplinarity, documentation, and scheduled review. This was supported by others (Grilli et al., 2000; Graham et al., 2000), and Heffner (1998) – in an early discussion of the influence of evidence-based medicine on clinical guidelines – proposed the following criteria: validity (will the guideline produce its intended health care outcomes?); reliability and reproducibility (would another groups of experts develop similar recommendations if provided with the same evidence?); clinical applicability, clarity, multidisciplinary process (including key stakeholders at various stages); scheduled review (for updates and revision); and documentation (an explicitly stated method for developing the guideline).

With the increasing interest in the implications of guideline development and use, several methodologies for the critical assessment of the quality of clinical guidelines have been developed (Shekelle et al., 1999; Vlayen et al., 2005; Lohr, 1994). Moreover, several studies of various aspects of clinical guidelines have been conducted. Burgers et al. – in their quest to identify and understand predictors of high-quality clinical practice guidelines – analysed 86 guidelines from 11 countries (of which 10 were European) and found that guidelines produced within a guideline programme and by governmental agencies scored better than their counterparts. Differences in the applicability of the guidelines could not be explained by the variables studied (Burgers, Cluzeau et al., 2003). Burgers also led a study to understand the structures and working methods of 18 major guideline programmes within and outside of Europe, and found that most guideline programmes explicitly aimed to improve the quality and effectiveness of health care, used electronic databases to collect evidence, conducted systematic reviews to analyse the evidence, and employed consensus procedures when evidence was lacking (Burgers, Grol et al., 2003b).

Vlayen et al. (2005) conducted a systematic review of tools to appraise clinical practice guidelines. They assessed 24 instruments developed between 1992 and 2003 from eight different countries. They and others since have concluded that the highest quality instrument overall is the widely employed and validated Appraisal of Guidelines for Research and Evaluation (AGREE) instrument (Delgado-Noguera et al., 2009; Vlayen et al., 2005; Burls, 2010).

AGREE

In 1998, the AGREE Collaboration was formed to coordinate guideline development internationally (Burgers, Grol et al., 2003a; AGREE Collaboration, 2003). Its work culminated in the publication of the now validated and widely used AGREE tool, which identified six quality domains and 23 specific items (Box 1.1). The six domains comprising the AGREE instrument are generally accepted to cover the key elements of the clinical guideline development process (AGREE Collaboration, 2003). AGREE II has since been developed

Box 1.1 *AGREE II domains*

Domain 1. Scope and purpose

1. The overall objective of the guideline is specifically described
2. The clinical question covered by the guideline is specifically described
3. Patients to whom the guideline is meant to be applied are specifically described

Domain 2. Stakeholder involvement

4. The guideline development group (GDG) includes individuals from all the relevant professional groups
5. Patients' views and preferences have been sought
6. The target users of the guideline are clearly described
7. The guideline has been piloted among target users

Domain 3. Rigour of development

8. Systematic methods were used to search for evidence
9. The criteria for selecting the evidence are clearly described
10. The methods used for formulating the recommendations are clearly described
11. The health benefits, side-effects and risks have been considered in formulating the recommendations
12. There is an explicit link between the recommendations and the supporting evidence
13. The guideline has been externally reviewed by experts prior to its publication
14. A procedure for updating the guideline is provided

Domain 4. Clarity and presentation

15. The recommendations are specific and unambiguous
16. The different options for management of conditions are clearly presented
17. Key recommendations are easily identifiable
18. The guideline is supported with tools for application

Domain 5. Applicability

19. The potential organizational barriers in applying the recommendations have been discussed
20. The potential cost implications of applying the recommendations have been considered
21. The guideline is supported with tools for application

Domain 6. Editorial independence

22. The guideline is editorially independent from the funding body
23. Conflicts of interest of guideline development members have been recorded

Source: AGREE Collaboration, 2010.

to refine the terms, improve supporting documentation, strengthen the tool's measurement properties, and test its utility for different stakeholders (Burls, 2010), and the AGREE Collaboration continues to develop instruments and toolkits (AGREE Collaboration, 2010).

Another evaluation strand focused on strategies to disseminate and implement clinical guidelines. The key assumption driving that research was (and still is): the more physicians know about guidelines, the more they will use them (and the better quality of care will become). Clearly, the most important question when evaluating clinical guidelines is: do clinical guidelines impact on the health of patients and the population; that is, do they change processes of care and ultimately patient outcomes? Grimshaw & Russell (1993) addressed this question and found that interest in clinical guidelines was increasing, but understanding whether they are effective had been hampered by the lack of a rigorous study. From their analysis of 59 published evaluations of clinical guidelines they concluded that explicit guidelines do improve clinical practice, when introduced in the context of rigorous evaluations. Since then, relatively few evaluation studies have addressed this important component. (See the systematic review of European country profiles in Part 6 of this report).

Grimshaw et al. followed up with their well-known study entitled *Effectiveness and efficiency of guideline dissemination and implementation strategies* (Grimshaw et al., 2004). They addressed questions such as "how do clinical guidelines reach their target audience?" and "what are the most successful implementation strategies?" They found considerable variation in the observed effects, both within and across interventions. Commonly evaluated single interventions included reminders, dissemination of educational materials, and audit and feedback. Multifaceted interventions included educational outreach. The majority of interventions observed modest to moderate improvements in care. The authors also sent out a survey to key informants from primary and secondary care settings to understand the feasibility and resource requirements of guideline dissemination and implementation strategies in the United Kingdom. Survey respondents reported that only dissemination of educational materials and short educational meetings would be feasible within the framework of existing resources.

Conceptual framework and methodology for the following sections

Conceptual framework

The brief review presented in the preceding section illustrates that there are different ways of defining clinical guidelines and how far these definitions go in establishing how clinical guidelines should be developed and who should be involved in the process. The following sections seek to understand how clinical guidelines are being developed and implemented across the EU, using a predefined conceptual framework, and the extent to which they comply with quality criteria; what means are being used to implement clinical guidelines and whether they have an impact on health outcomes. To achieve this it was necessary to begin by developing the conceptual framework (Fig. 1.2). This is described in more detail in the remainder of this section, and the findings are presented. Part 6 of the book applies this framework to examine how clinical guidelines have been developed and implemented in EU countries (plus Switzerland and Norway). The conceptual framework is also applied to each case study on type 2 diabetes mellitus and to the mapping exercise section. The conceptual framework consists of six dimensions: background; regulatory basis; development; quality control; implementation; and evaluation.

Background: this section describes whether clinical guidelines for preventing and/or treating chronic diseases exist in the country and, if they do not exist, whether there are other tools to assist professionals and patients in making appropriate decisions for patients with NCDs.

Regulatory basis: this section asks whether there is an "official" basis for clinical guideline development and implementation in the country; for example, a legal basis (possibly indirectly, as part of national service frameworks (NSFs) or Disease Management Programmes), a government document or a statement by an "arms-length" body (ALB) or quasi-official agency.

Development: this section asks whether the process of clinical guideline development is carried out centrally or whether is it decentralized; whether there are guidelines for clinical guidelines development (for example relating to the grading of evidence, stakeholder involvement, editorial independence), and by whom is this process coordinated.

Quality control: this section asks whether clinical guidelines are checked for quality (for example, using the AGREE instrument) before being implemented, and if so, by whom (that is, the same or a different body than those responsible for clinical guidelines).

Implementation: this section discusses whether the use of (certain) guidelines is mandatory (possibly with different terminology, such as "directives") or if there are financial incentives to implement and use clinical guidelines (for example, through contracts between purchasers and providers) and whether clinical guidelines are promoted through information technology (IT) applications.

Fig. 1.2 *Theoretical framework: clinical guidelines development, implementation and evaluation*

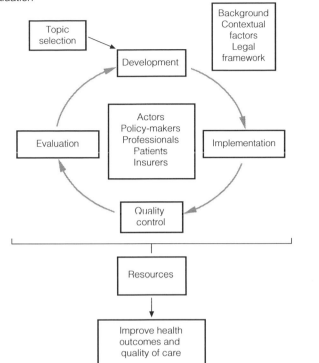

Source: Adapted from Council of Europe Recommendation Rec(2001)13 (Council of Europe, 2001).

Evaluation: this section asks whether the development, quality control, implementation and use of clinical guidelines (regularly) is evaluated, and if so, by whom.

Within the above conceptual framework, a particular focus was placed on identifying factors involved in guidance production. This was not only intended to provide a typology of developers but also to pinpoint key institutions in each country. Given both the multitude of clinical guideline definitions and the fact that the level of sophistication achieved by clinical guideline production mechanisms was expected to vary across countries, the framework specifically allowed for such factors to range from governmental institutions such as the ministries of health, to ALBs, to independent centres of excellence, to professional organizations and individual providers. In most cases more than one type of factor was identified, working either in collaboration or in parallel.

Methodology

The methodology of this report has been envisaged to provide information about how clinical guidelines on managing chronic conditions operate across the EU. Since very little is known about the topic, it is important to provide a general overview of how such guidelines function in each Member State. In order to collect this information a questionnaire was designed and sent to experts in the field of clinical guidelines. Mindful that this overview could be very general – perhaps overly so – the author team decided to focus on six Member States for a particular chronic condition, providing a thorough analysis to allow the reader to appreciate the complexities at a micro level. For this purpose, the questionnaire was developed on the management of type 2 diabetes mellitus and experts in the development and implementation of guidelines for this particular condition were contacted. The final step consisted of systematically reviewing the evidence on the development and effectiveness of clinical guidelines on chronic conditions in the EU. The rationale for this was that in many instances mapping exercises only describe what is being done but it is not possible to ascertain whether the resulting guidance is of high quality or has any effect. The two systematic reviews in this report aim to enrich the evidence in this respect, by providing a different type of information than the mapping exercise. All of these sources – once triangulated – provide a thorough overview of how clinical guidelines on the prevention and management of chronic conditions operate in the EU (Fig. 1.3).

Mapping exercise

This section provides an overview of how clinical guidelines are developed and implemented in Europe. Annex 2 provides a detailed profile for each country. Both sections follow the conceptual framework set out earlier. The profiles reflect the information that was available for collection. For some countries detailed information was gathered, while for others the information was scarce and difficult to obtain.

The information gathered on clinical guidelines can only be regarded as a first step. Attempts have been made to reduce or remove any inconsistencies in the accounts received by triangulating data from different sources, but some may remain.

The assessment of clinical guidelines in each country is based on three complementary sources: the book entitled *Assuring the quality of health in the European Union: a case for action* (Legido-Quigley et al., 2008), published by the European Observatory on Health Systems and Policies and written by several of the authors of this report; a review of the published and grey literature as identified through the systematic reviews and through the publications suggested by contributors; and information collected from key informants in each country by means of a questionnaire on clinical guidelines (see Part 6 of this report for the questionnaire template). In addition, in some cases

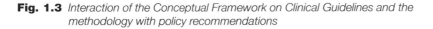

Fig. 1.3 *Interaction of the Conceptual Framework on Clinical Guidelines and the methodology with policy recommendations*

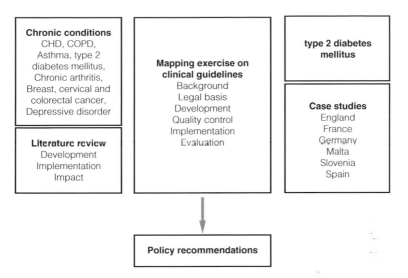

informants were asked further follow-up questions, telephone interviews took place and reviews of *Health Systems in Transition* series profiles were consulted.

The questionnaire was sent to experts on quality of health or the development and implementation of clinical guidelines in all countries, to associations of quality of care and to leading experts in the field of clinical guidelines in each country. Key experts in quality of health care with specialist knowledge of quality improvement were identified in all participating countries and there was at least one respondent for each country.

National "junior" representatives of general practitioner/family medicine organizations were also involved in the questionnaire through the United Kingdom representative of the Vasco da Gama movement, which is the European arm of the working group for new and future general practitioners associated with the World Organization of National Colleges, Academies and Academic Associations of General Practitioners/Family Physicians (WONCA). In several cases, the country representatives that were contacted forwarded the questionnaires to experts on clinical guideline development in their country. Thanks to this strategy and to the invaluable help of Luisa Pettigrew (United Kingdom representative) 17 responses were obtained.

The data collection process was conducted by e-mail. The total number of participants in the survey was 80: Austria (3), Belgium (7), Bulgaria (1), Cyprus (1), Czech Republic (1), Denmark (2), Estonia (2), Finland (3), France (3), Germany (2), Greece (2), Hungary (3), international (4), Ireland (1), Italy (3), Latvia (2), Lithuania (1), Luxembourg (3), Malta (6), Netherlands (2), Norway

(1), Poland (4), Portugal (3), Romania (3), Slovakia (3), Slovenia (2), Spain (6), Sweden (2), Switzerland (2) and the United Kingdom (England) (2).

A second stage of the research consisted of producing a profile for each Member State and sending this information to the country experts for feedback. This took place between February and May 2012. The purpose of this exercise was to resolve data inconsistencies and to incorporate recent changes in the field of clinical guideline development since the first phase of the research (September 2011).

In order to provide a more tangible foundation, six case studies were conducted, examining clinical guidelines for the prevention and treatment of type 2 diabetes mellitus. Countries were chosen specifically to include well-established clinical guideline programmes, as well as countries in which the development of guidelines is only beginning. Both centralized and decentralized systems were included to illustrate interactions between different actors and to provide examples of how processes can work in practice. A known case in which guideline development and implementation was not straightforward was also chosen in order to emphasize challenges inherent to guideline development. The methodological approach consisted of a questionnaire completed by experts on the development of type 2 diabetes mellitus guidelines (see the template in Annex 2), combined with utilization of relevant literature. This process was coordinated by a collaborator in each country.

Literature review

The aim of the literature review is to retrieve evidence on the quality of clinical guidelines developed in EU countries, as assessed by the AGREE criteria; the most effective strategies to disseminate and implement clinical guidelines; and the impact of the use of clinical guidelines on medical practice (processes) and patient outcomes. Three databases (Cochrane Central Register of Controlled Trials (CENTRAL), MEDLINE and EMBASE) were searched, applying the general search strategy presented in Annex 3, Table A3.1. Only studies published since 2000 and performed in EU countries were considered. Included studies focused on selected chronic conditions, in adults.[1] Different inclusion criteria were applied to select studies responding to the three main objectives of this research: development of clinical guidelines; dissemination and implementation of clinical guidelines; and impact of clinical guidelines (see Table 4.1 in Part 4 of the report).

---

1 CHD, COPD, asthma, type 2 diabetes mellitus, arthritis, breast cancer, cervical cancer, colorectal cancer, depressive disorder.

Part 2
Mapping clinical guidelines in Europe

H Legido-Quigley, D Panteli, C Knai, S Brusamento, U Augustin, V Saliba, M Solé, E Turk, M McKee and R Busse

This chapter provides a general overview of how clinical guidelines are developed, implemented and evaluated in Europe, applying the framework discussed in Part 1. Where possible examples are provided on the prevention and management of chronic conditions in particular, and Part 3 provides a more detailed analysis, discussing six case studies on type 2 diabetes mellitus.

Background

All countries within the EU are showing some interest in developing and implementing clinical guidelines. This is also an area of international cooperation, illustrated by projects such as the Council of Europe's Guideline Recommendation (Council of Europe, 2001), the EU-funded AGREE guideline research project (Burgers et al., 2004), and the Guidelines International Network (G-I-N), a Scottish charity coordinating the activities of national guideline agencies worldwide (Legido-Quigley et al., 2008). However, there is a great variability among countries. Most of them have an established clinical guideline programme, and a substantial proportion have developed clinical guidelines on preventing and/or treating chronic diseases, some within the framework of national programmes. Several countries have mechanisms in place to ensure transparency and scientific evidence is in the process of developing and using clinical guidelines, all with the aim of providing the highest possible quality of care, while others are increasingly interested in the development of guidelines and are making concerted efforts to establish systems that would allow their use. In addition, contributors to the mapping exercise reported the existence of other tools supporting professionals and patients with NCDs in decision-making processes, including continuing education (for example, self-management skills relevant to their disease), decision on supporting software and virtual networks. It has also been reported that hospitals are increasingly combining IT applications with clinical pathways based on clinical guidelines, although in most cases this development is still at an early stage, at least in the outpatient care setting.

Clinical guideline development has also been described at different levels of the system. In some cases the development is coordinated at a national level, but this can be adapted at regional or local levels. For example, the United Kingdom functions as four separate countries for this purpose, although with varying degrees of separation. In England, clinical guidelines are developed centrally through the National Institute for Health and Clinical Excellence (NICE), national collaborating centres (NCCs) and the Royal Colleges but may be adapted and implemented at the local level through hospitals, purchasers, local government, and non-governmental organizations. In other cases, for instance in Spain, the Clinical Practice Guideline Programme in the Spanish National Health System is coordinated by the Clinical Practice Guideline Library for the Spanish National Health System (GuíaSalud) (GuíaSalud, 2012a), which supervises guidelines production, with clinical guidelines being developed by HTA agencies and units from the different Autonomous Communities (Spanish regions), together with a pool of experts and Spanish medical societies and/or professional associations. Since the creation of the Clinical Practice Guideline Programme, they follow its methodological handbook for clinical guidelines development.

The existence of clinical guidelines for preventing and/or treating chronic diseases to some extent depends on how much of a priority this is for the individuals responsible for developing quality of care strategies and/or whether funds are available from governments to develop such programmes. The analysis of the country responses for this report distinguishes three broad categories of engagement in clinical guideline development. The first category includes those with "well-established" activities and with broad experience in the field of clinical guidelines. The second category includes those that have introduced some guidelines and are therefore "making progress" towards having adequate systems in place; and the third category involves those countries that have either "recently adopted" some clinical guidelines or where these are "in the planning stage" but some progress has been made in the conceptualization of how this might be operationalized in practice. There is no country in which no form of guidance for practitioners exists. In light of the increasing attention paid internationally to quality improvement, this is not a surprising finding. That said, certain countries still have a long way to go before clinical guidelines become established in mainstream clinical practice.

Countries with "well-established" activities

This category comprises the leaders in the development of guidelines (namely, Belgium, England, France, Germany and the Netherlands) and other countries that have well-established programmes (Finland, Norway and Sweden). All countries in this category have developed specific clinical guidelines for most diseases and especially for chronic diseases. In England, the NICE is the government-funded organization responsible for providing national guidance and setting quality standards for the promotion of good health and the prevention and treatment of ill health. The NICE produces guidance on public health, health technologies (pharmaceuticals, interventional procedures, devices and diagnostics) and clinical practice. It makes recommendations to the NHS, local authorities and other organizations in the public, private and voluntary sectors on new and existing medicines, treatments and procedures and on treating and caring for people with specific diseases and conditions. The NICE consults closely with independent committees and individual experts working in health care, academia and industry, as well as patients and members of the public with a background or interest in the area in question. The NCC for Chronic Conditions (NCCCC) – which is funded by the NICE and based at the Royal College of Physicians (RCP) – leads on developing clinical guidelines for the treatment of chronic conditions. The Centre for Public Health Excellence provides guidance on services that contribute to the prevention of chronic conditions and encourages good health and well-being.

In Germany, clinical guidelines are produced on a multitude of conditions, including the prevention and treatment of chronic diseases. The production of guidelines by professional associations is coordinated by their umbrella organization, the AWMF. Chronic diseases in particular are the focus of Disease Management Programmes (ÄZQ, 2010), which have been implemented nationwide by the statutory health insurance funds in recent years (for breast cancer and type 2 diabetes mellitus since 2002; for coronary heart disease and chronic heart failure due to coronary heart disease since 2003 and 2009, respectively; and for asthma and COPD since 2005). The utilization of indicators to promote quality assurance is not only an integral part of the national NVL programme but is also endorsed by other organizations, such as the Institute for Applied Quality Assurance and Research in Healthcare (AQUA Institute). In June 2011 the database of the AWMF contained 679 current guidelines (AWMF, 2012a). Guidelines are also collected by the German e-Health library, the Arztbibliothek (ÄZQ, 2011a).

The Netherlands also has a long tradition of producing clinical guidelines; they exist in both primary and specialist care, covering both prevention and treatment of NCDs. Sweden also has clinical guidelines covering both chronic and acute conditions (for example, diabetes, renal failure, coronary heart disease, cataract surgery, stroke, hip fracture and hip replacement, and malignant neoplasms). The same is true of Denmark, Italy and Norway.

Finland has national clinical guidelines covering over 100 clinical entities, many of them dealing with chronic conditions (such as diabetes, asthma, rheumatoid arthritis, and a range of malignant neoplasms). All cover treatment and most also extend to prevention. The clinical guidelines are used in developing regional care programmes. They are integrated with an Evidence-Based Medicine electronic Decision Support (EBMeDS) system, allowing clinical guidelines to be opened from within the electronic patient record.

In the Czech Republic, albeit with varying degrees of sophistication, over 250 clinical guidelines have been developed since 2006 and are periodically updated, including those covering diabetes, coronary heart disease, asthma/COPD and cancer. Several web portals exist to assist professionals and patients in making appropriate decisions but most are not systematically maintained.

In France, clinical guidelines are available on the web site of the French National Authority for Health (*Haute Autorité de Santé*, HAS) (HAS, 2010, 2012) or the web site of the Agency for the Safety of Health Products (*Agence française de sécurité sanitaire des produits de santé*, AFSSAPS), which is now under the National Security Agency of Medicines and Health Products (*Agence nationale de sécurité du médicament et des produits de santé*, ANSM) (ANSM, 2012).

In Spain, the Clinical Practice Guideline Programme within the National Health System (coordinated by GuíaSalud) was created in 2006. This national programme – established by ministerial agreement between the Spanish National Health System Quality Agency and HTA agencies and units – involved a commitment to draw up a common methodology for clinical practice guideline preparation, implementation and updating. The Clinical Practice Guideline Programme comprises 35 guidelines, representing an example of collaborations among regions, methodological consensus and allocation of tasks.

Countries "making progress" in the development of clinical guidelines

Some countries have clinical guidelines only for a few conditions, such as Luxembourg, where the *Conseil Scientifique* – comprising representatives of the Ministry of Health, the medical examination services department of the social insurance system, and associations of physicians and dentists – has published them on its web site for cardiovascular and cerebral diseases. Latvia has developed several guidelines, for example, for diabetes mellitus types 1 and 2, for COPD in primary care, for treatment of autoimmune inflammatory arthritis, for early detection of malignant tumours by general practitioners, and for palliative care and management of haemophilia.

In Hungary, clinical guidelines are produced by individual hospitals within a national framework. The national input comes from two newly created organizations, the National Advisory Board of Health Care (NABHC) and the National Institute for Quality and Organizational Development in Healthcare and Medicines (GYEMSZI), both established in 2011.

Malta has no national body charged with the task of developing and implementing clinical or public health guidelines; however, interested groups of clinicians have taken the initiative. Some of these guidelines cover the management of acute exacerbations of chronic diseases but none focus on prevention or long-term management. However, protocols for drug use exist that determine entitlement to government health services, developed by the Ministry's Medicines Entitlement Unit, some of which have characteristics of guidelines for chronic disease management.

It was not possible to identify a comprehensive suite of clinical guidelines in other countries, although individual practitioners or organizations may adopt international guidance, sometimes on an ad hoc basis, as is the case in Ireland. Examples include the symptomatic breast care standards and health care-associated infection standards. These guidelines have been mandated through the Health Information and Quality Authority (HIQA), a statutory body charged with regulating and inspecting health care services in Ireland. The Health Service Executive (HSE) is now rolling out a series of care specific programmes at national level, each with a clinical director and each specifically allocated the task of improving and standardizing care across health care services. Programmes exist for diabetes, stroke, acute medicine, elective surgery, and so on. Each programme will – as part of its activity – provide a specific set of guidelines agreed with clinical staff. These programmes are at an advanced stage of design and some are already being rolled out.

Some of the countries that are lacking guidelines have recognized the need to obtain them, at least as aspirations in national plans. In Poland the National Pharmaceutical Policy (2004–2008) published in 2003 identified a need for the development of ambulatory health care formularies (*receptariusz lecznictwa ambulatoryjnego*), which would contain guidelines on the use of medicines in specific cases and set standards of medical treatment, taking into account their costs. However, progress has been slow.

Countries "recently adopting" some guidelines or where these are "in the planning stage"

Several countries have recently adopted some guidelines or have begun to develop them. For example, in Slovenia, which lacks a comprehensive suite of clinical guidelines, practitioners may use international guidance on an ad hoc basis. The *Slovenian Medical Journal*, among others, has published various guidelines but their methodology is rarely stated. As there is no national responsible body, these guidelines are the product of groups of enthusiasts. The exception is a set of national guidelines and standards for diabetes, published as a comprehensive booklet (EndoDiab, 2012). However, the guidelines have not been authorized by the Health Council and their use remains optional.

In Greece, specialist medical societies have made recommendations for the management of diabetes, coronary heart disease, asthma/COPD (primary care) and rheumatoid arthritis. Clinical guidelines developed in other countries (mainly in English) are available on local medical societies' web sites. However, initiatives are not coordinated and individuals must themselves gather the evidence needed in order to make informed decisions.

Regulatory basis

The majority of countries have no legal basis for the development of clinical guidelines and those countries that have well-established systems have mostly decided to implement them on a voluntary basis. For example, in Germany, the AWMF – the umbrella organization of 158 medical societies – has been coordinating the development of clinical guidelines on behalf of the medical associations since 1995 (AWMF, 2012a). A separate type of guidelines, the NVL programme – which forms the basis for Disease Management Programmes – is coordinated by the AWMF, the German Medical Association (*Bundesärztekammer*, BÄK) in cooperation with the National Association of Statutory Health Insurance Physicians (*Kassenärztliche Bundesvereinigung*, KBV) via their joint institute, the German Agency for Quality in Medicine (*Ärztliches Zentrum für Qualität in der Medizin*, ÄZQ). These institutions agreed on national standards for guideline production and implementation based on Council of Europe Recommendation Rec(2001)13 (Council of Europe, 2001). The utilization of evidence-based guidelines is also firmly rooted in Social Security Statute V, which delineates the code of conduct for statutory health insurance.

In the Netherlands, too, many different organizations are involved, some with a regulatory function but others are based on professional norms. They include the National Institute for Public Health and the Environment (RIVM), the Dutch Institute for Healthcare Improvement (CBO), the Dutch Council for Quality of Care and the Dutch College of General Practitioners (NHG).

Only a few countries have some type of legal requirement to develop guidelines (such as in Hungary, Lithuania, the Netherlands and Sweden). The situation is different in France, for example, where the HAS has a statutory duty to publish clinical guidelines.[2] The same applies to the Directorate-General for Health (*Direcção-Geral da Saúde,* DGS) in Portugal, where clinical guidelines are also developed by the Portuguese Association of General and Family Medicine (APMGF).

Quality control

It is evident that countries with long-established processes for guideline production have systems to ensure their quality, although our conclusions are limited by a dearth of information. Having said that, the instrument developed by the AGREE Collaboration for evaluating the robustness of clinical guidelines has been generally well-accepted. Through the analysis of the responses to the questionnaires, it was possible to identify five distinctive categories: countries in which the AGREE instrument is widely used; countries in which there is no quality requirement but the AGREE instrument is often used; countries that are following an adapted version of AGREE; countries that are using other instruments; and, finally, countries in which no formal processes exist to assess the quality of clinical guidelines.

AGREE instrument widely used

In England, the guideline development process is based on the AGREE instrument (AGREE Collaboration, 2001) and described comprehensively in *The guidelines manual 2009* (NICE, 2009b). Stakeholder consultation, expert reviews and the assessment by the independent guideline review panel are all part of the validation process. Prior to publication the guidelines are subjected to an internal quality control assessment at the Centre for Clinical Practice. NHS Evidence accredits guidance producers, awarding them a seal of approval in the form of an Accreditation Mark. Guidelines are not piloted but are developed in a collaborative process with practitioners and service users. The independent guideline review panel also has a role in making sure that it will be feasible for the NHS to implement any recommendations. The ultimate test of the validity of NICE guidelines occurred during a judicial review in 2009 (NICE, 2009a). Litigation against the NICE was initiated by two patients with chronic fatigue syndrome/myalgic encephalomyelitis (CFS/ME) on the grounds of bias in the guideline development group (GDG) and its members; that the guideline was irrational compared to the evidence, and claims about the classification of the

---

2 Loi du 13 août 2004 relative à l'assurance maladie, Titre II, Chapitre Ier bis, article L. 161-37.

condition and treatments recommended. The High Court ruled in favour of the NICE on all allegations.

In Finland, prior to the completion of a guideline, it is circulated to interested groups for their critical consideration, according to the AGREE criteria. The Current Care Board selects the topics to be covered by clinical guidelines, mainly based on suggestions from specialist societies. These specialist societies operate as the host association for the guideline in question, in partnership with the Finnish Medical Society (Duodecim). The "PRIO-tool" – or a set of criteria for assessing the proposal – is used for prioritizing new guideline topics (Duodecim, 2011a). A systematic review of the literature on the topic is first conducted by an experienced information specialist. Current Care working groups (including approximately 700 volunteer health professionals from a range of fields across Finland) then produce the evidence-based clinical guidelines in cooperation with Current Care editors, who operate as methodological experts. Any resulting comments are then discussed and the guideline is revised if required. The completed clinical guidelines and subsequent updates are communicated as appropriate.

In the Czech Republic, the AGREE instrument is used by the Czech Medical Association of J.E.Purkyně.

In Norway, clinical guidelines are checked for quality using the AGREE instrument before being implemented. The AGREE instrument is used both during the development process and before implementation by the Secretariat of the Directorate of Health (Requirement) and the Norwegian Electronic Health Library before publishing the guideline online.

In Hungary, quality control of protocols is carried out by GYEMSZI. The AGREE instrument is used for quality assurance and the GYEMSZI is in the process of developing a methodological guide.

In Italy, quality assurance of clinical guidelines produced by certain bodies has been mandated by law since 1992, based on the AGREE instrument. The two organizations involved – the National Guideline System (SNLG) and the Centre for the Evaluation of the Effectiveness of Health Care (CeVeAs) – are responsible for this process, but there is also a dedicated agency responsible for quality control: the National Agency for Regional Healthcare Systems (AGENAS) (AGENAS, 2012a).

No quality requirement, AGREE instrument often used

Denmark has no formal requirement for quality assessment before implementation, but the AGREE instrument is often used in HTA.[3]

---

3 The Danish Centre for Health Technology Assessment (DACEHTA) is the main authority for HTA production in Denmark.

A similar situation has also occurred in Spain – there is a Clinical Practice Guideline Programme within the Spanish National Health System (GuíaSalud), along with informal use of the AGREE instrument. Belgium has no mandatory mechanisms for quality assurance and there is no widely used procedure in place. If requested, the Belgian Centre for Evidence-Based Medicine (CEBAM) will validate guidelines according to the AGREE instrument, with a limited analysis of the content. Sometimes this step is a prerequisite for funding care, for example for clinical guidelines proposed by the Belgian Health Care Knowledge Centre/Federal Centre of Health Care Expertise (KCE).

In Switzerland, the AGREE and ADAPTE instruments are used by some guidelines producers, such as the University of Lausanne.

Countries following an adapted version of AGREE

In Germany, guidelines coordinated by the ÄZQ or AWMF are checked for quality assurance before being implemented within the framework of the *Arztbibliothek*. The appraisal is carried out by means of the DELBI checklist (*Deutsches Instrument zur Bewertung der Methodischen Leitlinienqualität*, German Instrument for Methodological Guideline Appraisal) (ÄZQ, 2011b). The DELBI is based on the AGREE I instrument, adapted to the German context. The appraisal is performed by methodologists who were not part of the guideline production process. The AWMF categorizes guidelines according to their methodology using the so-called "S-classification" (*Stufenklassifikation von Leitlinien*),[4] with S1 being the lowest, drawing on expert opinion, and S3 being the highest, designating a guideline which is based on evidence and consensus process. In Ireland, in July 2011, the HIQA published draft guidance on quality criteria for clinical guidelines, which includes an adapted version of the AGREE II tool (HIQA, 2011).

Countries using other instruments

In France, the Guidelines Commission (Commission Recommendations) and the *College de la HAS* validate guidelines before they are published on their web sites. An evidence grading system is in use to assess the strength of evidence of each recommendation. The HAS model involves a GDG consisting of 15–20 specialists from different disciplines related to the topic, as well as representatives of health system users. The resulting recommendations are reviewed by a group of 30–50 people (with a composition similar to the GDG), which gives feedback about assessment to the GDG. The HAS seeks maximum transparency and objectivity through the independence of both groups.

---

4 S1: expert opinion-based; S2k: consensus-based; S2e: evidence-based; S3: evidence-based and consensus-based.

In the Netherlands, the methods used are different among organizations. In Austria, federal quality guidelines are subject to an explicit validation, while those developed by medical associations or expert groups are not. It is reported that the quality of clinical guidelines can vary quite significantly, depending on which medical society developed them. The only federal quality guideline that has been published so far on the web site of the Austrian Federal Ministry of Health (*Bundesministerium für Gesundheit*, BMG) is for type 2 diabetes mellitus (BMG, 2009). One issue of the journal *Guidelines,* published by the Medical Association of Upper Austria, has recommended a checklist for assessing the quality of guidelines (Alkin, 2001). Also, the web sites for Verlagshaus der Ärzte (Verlagshaus der Ärzte, 2012) and Arznei & Vernunft (Arznei & Vernunft, 2012) provide information on what are believed to be reliable guidelines for diagnoses and treatment pathways.

No formal processes to assess the quality of clinical guidelines

In Cyprus, there is no system of assessing clinical guidelines for their quality before being implemented, although this is being reviewed. In Lithuania, the development of clinical guidelines approved by the Ministry of Health involves consultation with Medical Faculties, the National Health Insurance Fund, the State Pharmaceutical Control Service and the Mandatory Health Insurance Service. Clinical guidelines developers are required to submit a draft before being reviewed by two particular national universities and subsequently by specific agencies of the Ministry of Health. However, it is not mandatory for the final version of the clinical guidelines to be approved by the Ministry of Health.

In Greece, there is no uniform process for quality control. In the development of the aforementioned clinical guidelines for diabetes, the American Diabetes Association (ADA) evaluation system and the Scottish Intercollegiate Guidelines Network (SIGN) evaluation system were used. For coronary heart disease, the European Society of Cardiology (ESCARDIO) Committee for Practice Guidelines (CPG) evaluation system has been used, and for asthma/COPD (in primary care), clinical guidelines use the International Primary Care Respiratory Group (IPCRG) evaluation system. The AGREE instrument is available (translated into Greek), but no evidence of its use was available for analysis for this report.

Development

Institutions and organizations responsible for developing clinical guidelines

The development of clinical guidelines across Europe varies according to which institutions are taking the lead and how decentralized the process is. In most countries, medical associations are involved in clinical guideline development, but their influence varies. In several cases, a central body (government or independent agency) is responsible for coordinating clinical guideline development. Three broad categories were identified: the first comprises those countries in which a national agency develops clinical guidelines; in the second category, multiple organizations contribute to the development of clinical guidelines, but central bodies coordinate the process; and the third category includes those countries in which professional associations are mostly responsible for clinical guideline development, with no central coordination.

Guidelines produced by a central agency

(In this group: England, Finland and Luxembourg)

While in several countries there is a main institution responsible for guideline production, only in three countries do national agencies exist that are entirely in charge of a top-down endorsement of recommendations. In England, the NICE produces guidance on public health, health technologies and clinical practice and makes recommendations to the NHS, local authorities and other organizations in the public, private and voluntary sectors. In Finland, the Current Care Editorial Office of the Duodecim is responsible for guideline production. Its *Käypä hoito* (Current Care) Unit drafts nationwide care guidelines to improve the quality of care and reduce variations in care practices. Finally, the Scientific Council has the key role for clinical guidelines in Luxembourg, consisting of members of the Ministry of Health, the medical examination services department of the social insurance system and various representatives of the associations of physicians and dentists.

Multiple actors are involved and there is a central component in place

(In this group: Austria, Cyprus, Czech Republic, Denmark, Estonia, France, Germany, Hungary, Italy, Latvia, Lithuania, Malta, Norway, Romania, Spain and Sweden)

This is a more heterogeneous group of countries, in terms of clinical guideline development mechanisms. The common characteristic is that while multiple institutions develop guidance, there is some level of central coordination of the entire process. This coordination may take different forms, as illustrated in the following examples. While in Norway the development of official national guidelines falls under the responsibility of the Directorate of Health, various professional associations produce their own guidance in parallel. A similar example is that of France, where the HAS is primarily responsible for central guidance production, but professional associations and sometimes regional authorities are also active in the field. Italy's SNLG supervises guidance production, but recommendations are also produced by medical societies and regional agencies. In Spain, the Clinical Practice Guideline Programme in the Spanish National Health System is coordinated by GuíaSalud, which supervises guidelines production, with the clinical guidelines being developed by HTA agencies and units from the different Autonomous Communities (regions), together with a pool of experts and Spanish medical societies and/or professional associations. The situation is similar in Denmark. In Germany, on the other hand, professional associations have their own umbrella organization, the AWMF, which coordinates guideline production. It further collaborates with other institutions to provide the evidence base for the NVL programme. In Hungary, overall directions are given by the NABHC, but providers can formulate their own specific guidance based on these directions; the implementation of these guidelines is subsequently monitored by the Board. In the Czech Republic, a governmental and a nongovernmental actor (the National Reference Centre and the DASHOFER publishing house, respectively) collaborate to produce clinical guidelines. In Austria, most guidelines are developed by professional associations, but an initiative is in place for national guidance, based on a contemporary meta-guideline approach.

Multiple actors produce guidance without central coordination

(In this group: Belgium, Bulgaria, Greece, Ireland, Netherlands, Poland, Portugal, Slovakia, Slovenia and Switzerland)

The commonality in this group of countries is that, while individual actors produce guidance, there is not one overarching agency or main institution playing a coordinating role. However, this is not indicative of the extent to which guidelines are developed: in Belgium, for example, several structures have been developed with the scope of disseminating the use of clinical guidelines, such as the colleges of physicians, the KCE, the CEBAM, the EBMPracticeNet (a voluntary platform of national evidence-based medicine organizations that aim to stimulate cooperation and coordination between the different actors) and the Federal Council for the Quality of Nursing. At the other end of the spectrum, practitioners in Greece need to rely to a great extent on their own efforts in order to obtain evidence, but some medical associations have begun to show interest in the field and to provide collected information or translations of international guidelines on their web sites. The Netherlands have a long and comprehensive tradition in terms of clinical guideline development, with a multitude of organizations active in the field, but in Poland guidance is generally produced sporadically, notably by the College of Family Physicians (CoPFiP). In Slovenia, guidelines have been produced by several types of institutions (professional associations, academic centres, and so on), as there is no national body responsible for clinical guidelines – instead, these are developed by groups of experts that have a professional interest in and enthusiasm for this field. In Ireland, multiple levers are in place to achieve quality assurance, but guidance is mostly used in an ad hoc manner and is usually taken from international literature.

Levels of operation

The way clinical guidelines are developed and implemented clearly also depends on the administrative organization of each country. Regional authorities may be informed by national recommendations, but the opposite process can also be observed; that is, national guidance synthesizing regionally developed information.

Local guidelines are based on centralized guidelines

In England clinical guidelines are developed centrally through the NICE, NCCs and the Royal Colleges, but may be adapted and implemented at the local level through NHS Hospital Trusts, Primary Care Trusts (PCTs), local authorities, or voluntary organizations. In Sweden, guidance produced by the National Board of Health and Welfare (NBHW) – an agency accountable to the Ministry of Health and Social Affairs – is usually adapted by counties and municipalities, which may also develop their own clinical guidelines.

Centralized guidelines are developed by regional agencies

In Spain, some clinical guidelines are elaborated within the Clinical Practice Guideline Programme in the Spanish National Health System (GuíaSalud). This guideline development process is commissioned by GuíaSalud for some institutions related to evidence-based medicine – mainly HTA units/agencies from different regions in Spain, following the national approach (as the guidelines are intended for use through the national programme). Afterwards, each Autonomous Community (region) may or may not adapt these guidelines to their regional or local context.

Implementation

The extent to which clinical guidelines are implemented in Europe is unknown, as there is no systematic data collection and, in most countries, no structure within which the data could be collected. In those few situations in which adherence to guidelines is mandatory, there is no systematic assessment of whether this has any effect. Hence, it is only possible to report what is meant to happen, rather than what actually takes place.

Mandatory and legal aspects

By definition, guidelines are just that, guidelines. Hence, their use can never be mandatory. However, there may be some legal requirement to take them into account, as in Hungary, Lithuania, the Netherlands and Sweden, in certain circumstances, such as end-of-life care in the Netherlands. In Hungary, providers are allowed to formulate clinical guidelines for their own setting based on the centrally issued protocols or recommendations, but are then obliged to implement their own formulations – a situation that precludes any meaningful monitoring. Similarly, in Italy, although clinical guidelines are optional, some mandatory protocols exist, mainly in the fields of occupational health and infectious disease control. Physicians enrolling in Disease Management Programmes in Germany are required to treat their patients according to the national guidelines (NVL programme). Also, whether or not treatment was carried out according to official guidelines can be used as an argument during malpractice cases.

Implementation aids

Many countries report that guidance is published online and thus made accessible to a wide audience, on the web sites of the agencies responsible for producing and disseminating them. In well-developed guidance systems, implementation is also aided by IT tools and other material. Most notably, the NICE has a team of implementation consultants that work nationally to encourage a supportive environment and to share learning and support education and training locally. Generic implementation tools exist, such as a "How to" guide and specific tools for every clinical guideline, such as a costing template and a PowerPoint presentation. Other tools may be produced jointly with organizations, such as professional or patient groups, and can include implementation advice to assist with action planning at an organizational level, referral letter templates, flow charts, fact sheets and checklists. In Sweden, several tools exist to facilitate the implementation and use of clinical guidelines, such as publications, educational material, conferences, IT applications, and even organizational interventions. Moreover, updated clinical guidelines are sent to each registered practitioner. In Finland, implementation is facilitated by linkage to medical records. In Belgium, an EBMeDS system is being implemented. It aims to bring evidence into practice by means of context-sensitive guidance at the point of care, through electronic patient records. In Portugal, IT tools are combined with specialized literature and specifically designed web sites. In Germany, indicator-based approaches are used to monitor and endorse implementation. Such tools may be forthcoming in countries in which the clinical guideline development system is still under development (such as in Cyprus).

Financial incentives

In some countries, such as Germany, Denmark and the United Kingdom, financial incentives are used to implement clinical guidelines (see the subsection on France within the case studies in Part 3).

Evaluation

There are few examples of formal evaluations of the development, quality, implementation and use of clinical guidelines. Some countries have made explicit efforts to address this question, while others are in the process of developing evaluation plans, and a third set has yet to consider the issue. The following subsections describe the clinical guidelines situation of European countries, according to the three broad groupings already described.

Formal evaluation of clinical guidelines

Several countries have reported evaluation processes, although these are not compulsory. For example, in Germany, although there is no national agenda on evaluating the implementation and use of guidelines, the National Academy of Family Physicians regularly evaluates all guidelines within its scope. The implementation and utilization of the national guidelines (NVL programme) are also evaluated in the clinical context of disease management contracts and in guideline-based quality indicator programmes.

In England, the NICE produces implementation reports, which measure the uptake of specific recommendations taken from selected pieces of guidance through the analysis of routine data. Interested researchers assess the uptake and effectiveness of guidance on an ad hoc basis. For example, a 2011 *British Medical Journal* article (Thornhill et al., 2011) demonstrates that, despite a 78.6% reduction in prescribing of antibiotic prophylaxis after the introduction of the related NICE guideline, the study excluded any large increase in the incidence of cases of or deaths from infective endocarditis in the two years after the guideline was implemented. Both kinds of report are collated by the NICE in a central, searchable database.

In Austria, the quality of federal guidelines has to be ensured by the responsible organization. Not only the guideline's impact on care quality, but also its acceptance and degree of implementation need to be evaluated. The reasons for any lack of implementation are required to be documented and analysed, and measures for improvement must be considered when reviewing the guideline. As far as possible, such evaluations should be representative and are to be carried out nationally. Funding for evaluation must be provided by the initiators of the guideline.

In Denmark, the development, quality control, implementation and use of clinical guidelines are evaluated within accreditation programmes for publicly funded hospitals. In Finland, clinical guidelines were not regularly evaluated until recently. However, since 2011, the National Institute for Health and Welfare (THL) (THL, 2012) has been responsible for supervising the development, quality and use of clinical guidelines.

In Norway, a draft of each of the national clinical guidelines must be sent for both internal and external evaluation/consultation. In the development of certain national clinical guidelines, an external "reference group" is also established to evaluate the process. There is usually an evaluation of clinical guidelines in connection with the revision process. The need for a revision of a national clinical guideline is expected to be considered within three years after the publication of the guideline.

In Sweden, the development, quality control, implementation and use of clinical guidelines are regularly evaluated by the NBHW (Socialstyrelsen, 2011).

In Italy, evaluation of clinical guideline adherence is required by law and the AGENAS is responsible for this. Reforms to introduce some kind of evaluation are currently under discussion.

There is no formal evaluation of clinical guidelines in Malta. In hospitals they are periodically evaluated by the Clinical Guideline Coordinating Committee (CGCC). In the primary care setting, no audits have been carried out as yet, but plans are under way for this to take place in the near future. In Cyprus, no evaluation processes are currently in place to evaluate the implementation and use of clinical guidelines. Tools for evaluating clinical guideline implementation have been proposed within the new National Health Insurance Scheme (NHIS). Similarly, in the Czech Republic, the evaluation of clinical guidelines is currently being developed. In Hungary, a partnership has been set up between the NABHC and the GYEMSZI to establish evaluation processes in the sector.

In Belgium no formal data currently exist on the extent to which clinical guidelines are used in the country. Generally, their use is not monitored, apart from for selected specific topics (such as antibiotics). A new system for the evaluation of hospital nursing clinical guidelines is being developed, from which initial results are expected in 2014. Some colleges of physicians also define criteria for clinical guidelines evaluations and assess them; however, this is not carried out systematically.

No formal evaluations of clinical guidelines

In the Netherlands, there is no official regulation for the evaluation of clinical guidelines. Individual research projects by scientific researchers, insurers or health professionals evaluate (methods of) quality control. In terms of implementation, there is still a lack of evaluation. However, several studies have been published to evaluate the implementation and impact of clinical guidelines (Frijling et al., 2002; Lub et al., 2006; Van Bruggen et al., 2008; Verstappen et al., 2003).

In France, the HAS clinical guideline methodology foresees that the agency should remain alert to developments so as to be able to initiate guideline updates if research emerges that suggests a significant deviation from existing recommendations. Given that guidelines are not mandatory, no official mechanism for evaluation is in place as yet.

In Greece, one study found that only 49% of Greek hospitals have any kind of practice guidelines for operating theatres, and of those only 51% applied them satisfactorily (see the Greek country profile in Part 6 of this report).

In Poland the monitoring of some aspects of implementation falls under the remit of the CoPFiP.

No evidence was available on the evaluation of clinical guidelines in Portugal, although it is reported that this is performed by a body within the DGS. However, the performance indicators used in the annual audit of family physician performance are being reviewed by the government contracting department (the ACSS).

In Spain, no impact evaluation is carried out formally; sometimes such evaluations are performed by the guideline developers, but there is still little experience in this field. However, the Spanish National Health System Quality Agency and some HTA agencies and units (regions) are rolling out a series of professional training programmes aiming to improve the quality of the guidelines. Moreover, the Clinical Practice Guideline Programme of the Spanish National Health System (GuíaSalud) has an implementation handbook (GuíaSalud, 2012c), which includes an evaluation chapter about the implementation process. The Spanish Ministry of Health is also funding a national project oriented towards assessing professionals' impressions relating to clinical guidelines. It is clear that the objectives regarding quality have been reasonably achieved and now implementation and impact evaluation are at the top of the Clinical Practice Guideline Programme agenda.

No evidence was available on the evaluation of the development, quality control, implementation and use of clinical guidelines in Ireland, Luxembourg, Slovakia, Slovenia or Switzerland.

Discussion

The mapping exercise illustrates the divergent status of clinical guideline production in the EU. A few countries have well-developed systems in place to develop clinical guidelines, while most have only fragmentary initiatives led by enthusiasts, with little more than aspirations to do something more formal at some unspecified time in the future.

The findings of this report on the value of a legal mandate are inconclusive. Spencer & Walshe (2009) suggested that having a legal requirement for quality improvement strategies was an important driver of progress. However, there are examples of laws that exist but are not implemented, as well as highly developed systems without any legal basis. Furthermore, legal measures may not always be appropriate to ensure compliance, illustrated by the fact that punitive provisions have been abandoned in France.

In general, guidelines are developed by government or quasi-governmental organizations and professional associations, often working together. A major factor is the motivation of individuals.

In the many countries without a comprehensive suite of clinical guidelines, individuals and organizations may rely on international guidance, either from pan-European or American bodies, or from other countries. For example, Slovakian practitioners seem to use Czech guidance. Some institutions, alongside their own clinical guideline programmes, also engage internationally with several networks established exactly for the purpose of knowledge exchange, methodological development and coordination of care. For example, in Germany the ÄZQ, the AWMF, the Federal Joint Committee (*Gemeinsamer Bundesausschuss*, G-BA), the Institute for Quality and Efficiency in Health Care (*Institut für Qualität und Wirtschaftlichkeit im Gesundheitswesen*, IQWiG) and several more institutions are members of the G-I-N.

Engaging stakeholders is a key feature in those countries with well-established clinical guideline systems. It is considered to be important to ensure transparency. Depending on the context, stakeholders can include representatives of professional organizations, service providers, the pharmaceutical industry and funding bodies; patients, their families and carers and patient representatives or organizations; academics or other experts; and/or other members of civil society. Their involvement in guidance production varies: for example, while the NICE consults registered stakeholders throughout the guideline development process, the HAS mostly involves them in the review of recommendations prepared by the GDG. The influence of pharmaceutical companies has rarely been reported by respondents to the questionnaires, although literature on this topic suggests that increasing contact has been reported between physicians and the pharmaceutical industry. As Choudhry and colleages suggest, these interactions are relevant since clinical guidelines are designed to influence the practices of a large number of physicians (Choudhry, Stelfox & Detsky, 2002). The French case study on the development of type 2 diabetes mellitus (see Part 3) highlights the importance of following a transparent process in guideline development.

Stakeholder involvement may also strengthen implementation, however, for example, NICE stakeholders are encouraged to use their networks and influence to encourage implementation of clinical guidelines at both national and local levels. However, overall, patient and service user organizations appear to have little influence on driving the development of clinical guidelines. Implementation can be facilitated by integration with IT systems, as is the case in the United Kingdom, Finland, Sweden and Germany (Kuchler et al., 2007). "NICE Pathways" is an online tool for health and social care professionals that brings together all related NICE guidance and associated products in a set of interactive topic-based diagrams (NICE Pathways, 2011).

Those organizations seeking to ascertain the quality of their guidelines use the AGREE instrument, in some cases adapted to context, while others have developed their own approaches. Overall, the AGREE instrument seems to be well-accepted among participating countries, although there are many reports of countries in which no formal processes to assess the quality of clinical guidelines exist. Willingness to devote resources to this area seems to be important in determining systems to develop and evaluate clinical guidelines. The most appropriate model for clinical guideline implementation varies according to the setting. There is also a need to produce costing reports that estimate the national savings and costs associated with implementation and a costing template that can be used to estimate the local costs and savings involved. Similarly, when exploring how countries evaluate clinical guidelines, although some countries have made explicit efforts to address this question, most countries do not have any formal way to regularly evaluate the development, quality control, implementation and use of the guidelines.

This mapping exercise provides an updated and thorough overview of how clinical guidelines operate in Europe. A limitation of this exercise is that, while the authors were able to collect information on all included countries, this information is quite general and it does not allow important aspects of clinical guidelines development to be ascertained, such as the barriers to implementation, their impact and whether those guidelines that are being developed are of good quality. Once again, there is a lamentable lack of information on the basic aspects of clinical practice in many European countries, with no effective system for exchanging information other than ad hoc exercises, such as this one. This ignorance raises serious questions about how it is possible to enact European legislation on health care provision, such as that relating to the cross-border movement of health professionals. The following sections of this report discuss these important issues. First, a detailed analysis of guideline development is provided, by means of a case study of a specific condition (type 2 diabetes mellitus), followed by a presentation of the findings of three reviews on the evidence available relating to the development, dissemination and implementation – as well as impact – of clinical guidelines in European countries.

Part 3

Case studies on clinical guidelines for the prevention and treatment of type 2 diabetes mellitus

D Panteli, H Legido-Quigley, V Saliba, C Knai, M Solé, E Turk,
M McKee and R Busse

Introduction

As mentioned earlier, the mapping exercise provides an updated and thorough overview of how clinical guidelines operate in Europe. However, a limitation of this exercise is that, while information was collected on all included countries, it is quite general and broad based. This section attempts to fill this gap by illustrating in greater detail the commonalities and differences in clinical guidelines development, implementation and evaluation across participating countries, as exemplified by six case studies on clinical guidelines for the prevention and treatment of type 2 diabetes mellitus. The selection of countries aimed to capture the spectrum of development pinpointed by the mapping exercise, thus including well-established clinical guidelines programmes alongside countries in which the development of guidelines is only beginning. Additionally, both centralized and decentralized systems are included in order to illustrate interactions between different actors. Finally, a known example (France) where there have been instances when the process of guidelines was not straightforward was intentionally included to emphasize the challenges involved in clinical guideline development. Each case study is presented individually according to the framework developed for this research, followed by a short discussion to showcase commonalities and differences in practice (see Chapter 1).

United Kingdom (England)

Background, policy context and regulatory basis

This case study is focused on England, recognizing that other parts of the United Kingdom (such as Scotland) also have well-established clinical guidelines programmes. The SIGN – formed in 1993 – develops evidence-based clinical practice guidelines for the NHS in Scotland. SIGN guidelines are derived from a systematic review of the scientific literature and developed by multidisciplinary working groups (SIGN, 2012). They are regarded as being exemplary internationally and several countries, such as Austria, Greece and Malta, have been influenced by their methodological guidance.

In England, the NSF for Diabetes (Department of Health, 2001) set out a 10-year programme of change to deliver world-class care and support for people with diabetes. It included standards, rationales, key interventions and an analysis of the implications for planning services. This was the first-ever set of national standards aimed at developing a patient-centred service and improving health outcomes for people with diabetes in England, raising the quality of services and reducing unacceptable variations between them. Ten years later, NICE published a "quality standard for diabetes" (NICE, 2011a), which supports the existing NSF and provides an authoritative definition of high-quality care.

The NICE *Diabetes in Adults Quality Standard* defines clinical best practice within this topic area. It provides specific, concise quality statements, measures and audience descriptors to provide patients and the public, health and social care professionals, commissioners and service providers with definitions of high-quality care. It requires that services should be commissioned from and coordinated across all relevant agencies, encompassing the whole diabetes care pathway.

Development and implementation

The type 2 diabetes mellitus clinical guidelines were developed by the NCCCC, the Centre for Clinical Practice, the Centre for Public Health Excellence and the Centre for Health Technology Evaluation at the NICE. In England, clinical guidelines are generally developed centrally through the NICE, NCCs and the Royal Colleges, but may be adapted and implemented at the local level through NHS Hospital Trusts, PCTs, local authorities and voluntary organizations. The steps of the guideline development process can be seen in Box 3.1.

Box 3.1 *Guideline development process for the NICE clinical guidelines on diabetes*

Guideline topic is referred. The Department of Health, acting on behalf of the Secretary of State for Health commissions the National Institute for Health and Clinical Excellence (NICE) to develop clinical guidelines (CGs) on a particular topic. Normally topics are chosen due to confusion or uncertainty among health care professionals about the value of a drug, device or treatment, for example.

Stakeholders register interest. National organizations, representing patients, carers, and health professionals involved in their care, can register as stakeholders. Stakeholders are consulted throughout the guideline development process. In the field of diabetes, stakeholders include the Association of British Clinical Dialectologists, the British Dietetic Association, Diabetes UK, the Institute for Innovation and Improvement Think Glucose Campaign, the National Diabetes Information Service, NHS Diabetes, the Primary Care Diabetes Society, the NHS Retinal Screening Programme and the Royal College of Nursing. About 200 registered stakeholders were involved in the development of the public health diabetes guidance (NICE, 2011c).

Scoping. The National Collaborating Centre (NCC), commissioned to develop the guideline prepares the scope. This document sets out what the guideline will and will not cover. The NICE, registered stakeholders and an independent guideline review panel can all contribute to the development of the scope.

Guideline development group (GDG) is established. The NCC sets up an independent GDG for each clinical guidelines being developed. Group members include health professionals and patient/carer representatives with relevant expertise and experience.

Draft guideline is produced. To produce the draft guideline, the group assesses the available evidence and makes recommendations.

Consultation on the draft guideline. There is at least one public consultation period for registered stakeholders to comment on the draft guideline. During this time the NICE commissions expert peer reviewers to carry out a statistical and health economics review of each CG.

Final guideline produced. After the GDG finalizes the recommendations, the collaborating centre produces the final CG.

Over the years NICE has produced more than 10 clinical guidelines relevant to type 2 diabetes mellitus prevention and management for England and Wales. These have included clinical guidelines related to the treatment of type 2 diabetes mellitus (e.g. on managing blood glucose levels), diabetic foot care, diabetic renal disease and retinopathy. In May 2011 NICE issued public health guidance on the prevention of type 2 diabetes mellitus, focusing on population and community interventions. There are also a number of diabetes-related appraisals, such as the appraisal on treatment with liraglutide. New guidelines and appraisals are continuously being developed – there are currently about 10 in progress for type 2 diabetes mellitus. There is a formal process for reviewing and updating clinical guidelines, which follows a three-year cycle but a partial update may also be carried out earlier if significant new evidence emerges.

All guidelines are widely available online through the NICE web site. The relevant Royal Colleges also have electronic links to guidelines through their web sites. NICE produces different versions of the guidelines. The full version contains all the background details and evidence for the guideline, as well as the recommendations. This document is produced by whichever NCC is responsible for the guideline. The "NICE Guideline" contains only the recommendations from the full guideline, without the information on methods and evidence. The quick reference guide summarizes the recommendations in an easy-to-use format for health care professionals. In each case, the version entitled "Understanding NICE guidance" summarizes the recommendations in plain language and is aimed at patients and their families and carers.

Diabetes guidelines have also been incorporated into the Diabetes NICE Pathways (NICE Pathways, 2011), along with related guidance and products. NICE Pathways are an online tool for health and social care professionals, bringing together all related NICE guidance and associated products in a set of interactive topic-based diagrams. Visually representing everything the NICE has said on a particular topic, NICE Pathways presents at a glance all of the NICE's recommendations on a specific clinical or health topic. They provide an easier and more intuitive way to access and use NICE guidance.

NICE clinical guidelines are advisory rather than compulsory, but the NHS considers that they should be taken into account by health care professionals when planning care for individual patients. The type 2 diabetes mellitus guidelines apply to all patients with that specific condition, but there will be times when the recommendations are not appropriate for a particular patient. In any case, guidance is not supposed to override clinicians' responsibility to make decisions appropriate to the circumstances of each patient. These decisions should be made in consultation with, and with the agreement of, the patient and/or their guardian or carer. However, health care professionals are expected to record their reasons for not following clinical guideline recommendations.

NICE supports the implementation of its guidance by engaging stakeholders, patients and the public in the selection of topics and in the guidance development process. Stakeholders are encouraged to use their networks and influence to advance the implementation of the clinical guidelines at both national and local levels. NICE develops and uploads onto its web site a range of tools to help the NHS in implementing clinical guidelines (see Chapter 6 for more details).

It also produces implementation reports that provide information on national trends and activity associated with recommendations in NICE guidance. These reports, along with other, both internal and external literature sources – often ad hoc studies led by interested researchers in the field – relating to the uptake of NICE guidance are stored on and can be accessed from the Evaluation and Review of NICE Implementation Evidence (ERNIE) database. Table 3.1 summarizes the results of a search on the database to find reports on the implementation of type 2 diabetes mellitus guidelines.

Table 3.1 *ERNIE search: type 2 diabetes mellitus*

Reference	Title	NICE implementation uptake reports	External literature
TA63	Diabetes (type 2) – glitazones (replaced by Clinical guideline 66)	0	2
TA53	Diabetes (types 1 and 2) – long acting insulin analogues	0	1
TA60	Diabetes (types 1 and 2) – patient education models	0	2
Clinical guideline 63	Diabetes in pregnancy	0	3
Clinical guideline 55	Intrapartum care	0	3
Clinical guideline 67	Lipid modification	0	1
TA46	Obesity (morbid) – surgery (replaced by Clinical guideline 43)	0	1
TA22	Obesity – orlistat (replaced by Clinical guideline 43)	0	5
Clinical guideline 66	Type 2 diabetes (partially updated by Clinical guideline 87)	2	2
G	Type 2 diabetes – blood glucose (replaced by Clinical guideline 66)	0	2
Clinical guideline 10	Type 2 diabetes – footcare	0	1
Clinical guideline 87	Type 2 diabetes – newer agents (partial update of Clinical guideline 66)	0	4

Source: Authors' search on ERNIE, September 2011 (NICE, 2012b).

Quality control and evaluation

In March 2011 NICE published an implementation report on the management of type 2 diabetes (NICE, 2011b), which covered the monitoring and control of glucose, lipid and blood pressure levels using medication, diabetes education programmes and dietary advice. It also covered the detection and ongoing management of eye disease, kidney disease, nerve damage and nerve pain.

Germany

Background, policy context and regulatory basis

Germany has a long tradition in the development of clinical practice guidelines and an increasing awareness of the need to monitor the quality and implementation of existing guidelines. Guideline development is coordinated by the AWMF, which maintains a guideline database and is, together with the ÄZQ (a joint subsidiary of the BÄK and the KBV), responsible for the NVL programme, which deals primarily with the conditions for which Disease Management Programmes exist (see chapters 2 and 6 for more information). Agreements (*Vereinbarungen*) on the establishment of Disease Management Programmes are forged between the Associations of Statutory Health Insurance Physicians (*kassenärztliche Vereinigungen*), the corresponding regional branches of health insurance funds and some hospitals at federal state (*Länd*) level. Such agreements for type 2 diabetes mellitus exist in all federal states (*Länder*). The type 2 diabetes mellitus Disease Management Programme – launched nationwide in 2003 – encompasses all aspects of care relevant to the condition, including diagnostics, therapeutics, the consideration of co-morbidities, the prevention of complications and rehabilitation, and the coordination of different levels of care and providers. The Disease Management Programme aims primarily at increasing life expectancy and health-related quality of life. Participation is voluntary for physicians and patients but financial incentives are provided by Sickness Funds. Once enrolled in the Disease Management Programme, the physician is obligated to treat the patient according to the provisions of the programme and to join quality improvement networks in order to exchange information with other professionals in the programme. The German Federal Insurance Authority reported that 64% of type 2 diabetes mellitus patients with statutory health insurance (estimated at about 5million) were enrolled in the programme in August 2009. Studies evaluating the programme have shown that it enjoys increased acceptance on behalf of the patients and improves the process quality of diabetes care (Schafer et al., 2010). However, acceptance and, consequently, drop-out levels show regional variation, as some federal states have had similar structures in place for longer periods than others.

OECD data indicate that 12% of the German population between the ages of 20 and 79 years were affected by type 2 diabetes mellitus in 2010. Given the complex nature of the condition, guidelines on its treatment and the prevention and treatment of its complications are produced by the German Diabetes Association (*Deutsche Diabetes-Gesellschaft*, DDG) in cooperation with other medical associations, and coordinated by the AWMF. There is also a national guideline on type 2 diabetes mellitus consisting of different modules (see the subsections that follow). All valid diabetes-related guidelines can be found online within the AWMF database, with additional documents available from the DDG web site (DDG, 2012). The ÄZQ also maintains its own portal for guidelines research (AWMF, 2012a). As of 2008, all evidence-based guidelines produced by the DDG are to be updated within the framework of the NVL programme.

In 2009, the G-BA commissioned the IQWiG to systematically research and evaluate existing guidelines on type 2 diabetes mellitus in order to ensure the validity of requirements of the type 2 diabetes mellitus Disease Management Programme [Annex 1 of the Risk Adjustment Act (German Federal Law Gazette, 1994)]. The report was officially published in January 2012 and is available in German from the IQWiG web site (IQWiG, 2011).

Development and implementation

Medical associations – the DDG

Individual guidelines on type 2 diabetes mellitus are produced by the DDG, which is also a member of the AWMF and contributes to the national guidelines. The DDG encompasses several committees (*Ausschüsse*) and consortia (*Arbeitsgemeinschaften*) that are responsible for various diabetes-related disciplines (such as pharmacotherapy, nutrition and psychology). Depending on the guidance topic, the Board and the Guideline Commission of the DDG choose the appropriate multidisciplinary development group and recruit external experts to provide additional evidence and enhance transparency. Literature reviews are undertaken in MEDLINE, the Cochrane Library and EMBASE by the GDG, once the search terms have been agreed on with the experts. Each guideline includes an annex with the search strategy and terms. The retrieved evidence is assessed on the basis of Agency for Health Care Policy and Research and SIGN classifications (both in terms of level of evidence and grade of recommendation). Consensus is based on discussion. Guidance drafts are published on the DDG web site for a specific amount of time and are thus made available for feedback to a wide audience, including patients and patient organizations. Feedback provided within the specified time frame is considered in full by the GDG and the external experts, who then incorporate it in the final guideline version. The DDG publishes two types of guidelines on its web site: evidence-based guidelines, which synthesize and grade existing evidence and provide recommendations, and practice guidelines, which operationalize the aforementioned recommendations and provide algorithms to facilitate utilization. It also provides patient information and guidance materials. The DDG guidance is financed by the DDG itself. DDG Regional Societies (*Regionalgesellschaften*) – which are the representatives of the Association at federal state level – are responsible for the realization of the Association's roles within their catchment area; part of this responsibility involves the evaluation of guideline implementation.

Given the nature of the condition, other medical associations may include recommendations for diabetes in their own guidance. Guideline production and cooperation is coordinated by the AWMF and all guidance is available on the AWMF database (AWMF, 2012a). The guidelines manual available on the AWMF web site provides methodological support for medical associations producing guidelines, including the DDG (AWMF & ÄZQ, 2000). The AWMF also uploads related publications that can be helpful both for guideline developers and users.

NVL programme

The AWMF, BÄK and KBV launched the NVL programme in 2002 to provide the scientific infrastructure for the German Disease Management Programmes (DMPs). All activities related to the programme are financed by these three institutions and are coordinated and administrated by the ÄZQ. The NVL programme has its own methodological handbook, which summarizes the guideline production process (AWMF, BÄK & KBV, 2010). NVL GDGs put recommendations together by systematically researching and synthesizing existing guidance, publications with aggregated evidence in the form of systematic reviews, meta-analyses and HTA reports, as well as primary literature. GDGs are multidisciplinary, including experts from the medical associations participating in the AWMF, patient representatives and potentially representatives from other associations (for example, for physiotherapy, ergotherapy and so on). Retrieved material is assessed regarding both level of evidence and grade of recommendation, and consensus on recommendations to be included in the national guidelines is reached by means of the Delphi method. Guidelines are given a pre-specified validity time frame and are assessed six months before their expiration to determine the need for updates. At the same time, two processes for the continuous identification of new relevant publications are in place (University of Bremen, ÄZQ). All guidelines are published upon completion on the NVL web site and the AWMF and G-I-N databases. The first edition of the TD2M NVL was published in 2002.

Modular updates to the guideline were initiated in 2006.[5] Furthermore, the ÄZQ, the AWMF, the G-BA, the IQWG and several more institutions in Germany are members of the G-I-N (G-I-N, 2012).

In principle, diabetes guidelines are not mandatory in Germany. As mentioned above, financial incentives for their use exist, within the DMPs. Tools based on quality indicators are endorsed by the NVL programme, in order both to endorse and to enhance national guidelines (ÄZQ, 2009). Clinical pathways based on guidelines are being used increasingly in hospitals in Germany and proposals for diabetes pathways have been made (Kuchler et al., 2007).

Quality control and evaluation

As mentioned earlier, the DDG and the NVL programme use both the level of evidence and the grade of recommendation to evaluate data found in the retrieved material. The NVL programme and the *Arztbibliothek* (ÄZQ, 2011a) use the DELBI tool (ÄZQ, 2011b), which is based on AGREE I and has been contextualized for Germany. The IQWiG uses the AGREE II instrument to ascertain whether published guidelines are robust enough to be taken into account when updating the regulation on Disease Management Programmes. The AWMF uses the so-called S-classification to categorize guidelines with regard to their methodological consistency (with S1 being the lowest, drawing on expert opinion, and S3 being the highest, designating a guideline which is based on evidence- and consensus-based).

Updates are organized by the AWMF for guidelines produced by the medical associations and the G-BA is responsible for updating the regulations behind Disease Management Programmes (as mentioned earlier, the related scientific research in the case of type 2 diabetes mellitus has been undertaken by the IQWiG). There are no fixed intervals for re-evaluation or update.

Table 3.2 shows a list of currently valid guidelines on type 2 diabetes mellitus along with their S-classification, as retrieved from the AWMF database in September 2011.

---

5 All information is available at the NVL Programme web site, operated by the ÄZQ (ÄZQ, 2012).

Table 3.2 *Valid guidelines on type 2 diabetes mellitus from the AWMF database in September 2011*

Title	Classification	Valid until
DDG guidance		
Supervision of neonates with diabetic mothers	S2k	31 May 2015
Obesity treatment for children and adolescents	S3	1 January 2012
Nutrition recommendations for the treatment and prevention of diabetes mellitus	S2	1 June 2015
Pharmaceutical antihyperglycaemic treatment for type 2 diabetes	S3	1 October 2013
Diagnostics, treatment and follow-up of diabetes mellitus in children and adolescents	S3	1 April 2013
Activity and diabetes mellitus	S3	1 October 2013
Diabetes and pregnancy	S3	30 April 2014
Relevant guidance of other associations		
Parenteral nutrition	S3	1 April 2014
Histopathological diagnosis of non-alcoholic and alcoholic fatty liver disease	S2k	1 November 2014
Modules of the NVL guidance		
NVL Type-2-Diabetes: Prevention and treatment of retinal complications	S3	30.09.2011
NVL Type-2-Diabetes: Prevention and treatment strategies for diabetic foot syndrome	S3	31.10.2011
NVL Type-2-Diabetes: Kidney disease in diabetic adults	S3	01.102014
NVL Chronic Heart Failure	S3	01.12.2013

Source: Authors' search on the AWMF database, September 2011 (AWMF, 2012b).

The acceptance of clinical guidelines on different levels has been a matter of interest in recent years and barriers have been identified in general care (Bolter et al., 2010; Ollenschläger, 2007; Hasenbein, Wallesch & Räbiger, 2003) and for the diabetes Disease Management Programme (Schafer et al., 2010; Nagel, Baehring & Scherbaum, 2006).

France

Background, policy context and regulatory basis

The Haute Authorité de Sauté (HAS) develops, finances and publishes national evidence-based clinical guidelines (HAS, 2012). This can be carried out in partnership with professional associations and medical societies; in this event, the HAS coordinates the work according to its defined clinical guideline development method. Guidelines developed by external agencies follow the development method established by the HAS, but without financial support from the institution. The HAS then provides methodological support and analyses the work using the AGREE II method. If the methodological quality of the guideline is satisfactory, HAS might then officially let the guideline be issued under its auspice. However, the HAS is not responsible for the content of the literature and recommendations (see chapters 2 and 6 for more information).

The most recent (2006) HAS guideline on type 2 diabetes mellitus was officially retracted by the HAS on 2 May 2011 because public statements declaring potential conflicts of interest between certain parties in the original 2003 guideline working group could not be produced (HAS, 2011). A working group established by the HAS to develop the updated clinical guideline conformed to the latest rules for managing conflicts of interest. A "scoping memorandum" or plan for the development and implementation of the "Medical treatment strategy of glycaemic control for type 2 diabetes" has been prepared, describing the draft recommendations which will inform the new clinical guideline. The 2006 recommendations are being updated on two specific points: glycaemic targets and medical treatment. The target population for the new guideline is adult patients with type 2 diabetes mellitus; the target health professionals are general practitioners, diabetologists and other endocrinologists, nurses, and other health professionals supporting patients with diabetes. The updated clinical guideline was issued in February 2012.

Additional tools to assist professionals and patients in making appropriate decisions on chronic conditions such as type 2 diabetes mellitus are the "ALD Guides" (*affectations de longue durée* or long-term conditions). The ALD scheme, based on a list of 30 (mostly chronic) diseases, aims to protect those with long-term conditions from financial hardship associated with disease. An ALD guide for type 2 diabetes mellitus[6] explains to medical health professionals the optimal management and care pathway of a patient admitted under the ALD system (Chevreul et al., 2010). This is currently being reviewed to become a more comprehensive type of guideline that will address the entirety of the condition and is expected to be finalized by the end of 2013. ALD guides – versions for health care professionals and for patients – are sent to general practitioner offices and hospitals. Patients are encouraged by their health insurer to join the ALD system and participation is free of charge. General practitioners are invited directly by the health insurer to follow up with the patient and to meet the ALD programme objectives; participating general practitioners receive €66 per patient per year (Chevreul et al., forthcoming).

Development and implementation

Type 2 diabetes mellitus guidelines have been developed in accordance with the method established for evidence-based clinical guidelines by the

---

6 footnote ALD No. 8 – Diabète de type 2 – 31 May 2006.

HAS. This involves two groups of active participants over four phases. A multidisciplinary working group is established by the HAS, comprising 15–20 health professionals and patient representatives, and is led by a chairperson, a HAS project manager and a project officer. The working group does not undergo specific methodological training; however, guideline development guides are available to provide methodological support (HAS, 2010). The working group members must have a good knowledge of professional practice in the field and be capable of assessing the relevance of the published studies and the various clinical situations evaluated. The project officer leads the systematic review of the literature, which is summarized in an evidence report along with the recommendations. In the absence of evidence, suggested recommendations will appear in the text of the guideline submitted to the peer review group if they receive the approval of at least 80% of the working group's members, and will constitute "expert consensus". The evidence report is then submitted to an external peer review group, comprising 30–50 health professionals, patient representatives, medical specialists and civil society members both included and not included in the working group. Individual opinions are given on the content and form of the initial version of the guideline, in particular its applicability, acceptability and readability. After the external peer review phase, the working group finalizes the recommendations according to the peer review group's assessments and comments.

The use of clinical guidelines is not mandatory. However, especially in the case of type 2 diabetes mellitus, the *Programme d'évolution des pratiques* (CAPI) scheme acts as an indirect incentive for the use of clinical guidelines. The 2009 Social Security Financing Act (SSFA) introduced the CAPI scheme, which aims to improve the quality and efficiency of care and to complement the prevailing fee-for-service remuneration by introducing a pay-for-performance model (Chevreul et al., 2010; Chevreul et al., forthcoming). The CAPI consists of voluntary individual contracts between general practitioners and the statutory health insurance (*assurance maladie*), whereby the general practitioner agrees to meet specific objectives relative to chronic diseases management and treatment. One of the main objectives of CAPI contracts is to improve the proportion of diabetic patients treated in line with current recommendations put forth in the national diabetes clinical guidelines (Chevreul et al., 2010). Specifically, the CAPI provides benchmarks regarding medical practice, based on evidence-based performance indicators for prevention and monitoring of chronic conditions (L'Assurance Maladie, 2010). Of the performance measures for chronic disease included in the CAPI, four are related to diabetes (HbA1c check, ophthalmologist check-up, use of low-dose aspirin and use of statins), in line with the French clinical guidelines developed by the HAS. Thus, there is an indirect financial incentive for guideline adherence, even though it is not imposed by the HAS.

New or updated clinical guidelines are disseminated to health care providers via direct mailing and via the HAS web site. This is supplemented by scientific publications and conference presentations that may involve members of the working group.

Quality control and evaluation

The final document is sent to a committee for the validation of clinical guidelines. Quality control includes appraisal using the AGREE tool. Once the committee has signed off the guideline, it is sent to the HAS Board for official validation, production and dissemination. The HAS Board is the deliberative body of the HAS, and is responsible for ensuring the rigour and impartiality of HAS products, including the clinical guidelines.

Malta

Background, policy context and regulatory basis

The first national Strategy for the Prevention and Control of Noncommunicable Disease was published in 2010 by the Department of Health Promotion and Disease Prevention of the Ministry of Health, the Elderly and Community Care. The Strategy was an attempt by the Government to shift its focus from treatment and curative services to prevention services. It identifies the development and implementation of national evidence-based guidelines on the primary and secondary prevention of NCDs as a priority for action (Department of Health Promotion and Disease Prevention, 2010).

There is no national body responsible for developing and implementing clinical and public health guidelines in Malta. Interested groups of clinicians working in primary and secondary care have developed clinical practice guidelines for use within their own departments. Some of these guidelines cover the management of acute exacerbations of chronic diseases, but none focuses on their prevention or long-term management of chronic diseases. Medicine protocols used for entitlement purposes within the Government Health Services are developed and implemented nationally by the Medicines Entitlement Unit and some of these cover medicines used in the treatment of chronic diseases such as type 2 diabetes mellitus.

Implementation and evaluation

The guidelines are endorsed by the Primary Health Department but are not mandatory, so health care professionals are free to use them based on their own clinical discretion. The clinical guidelines are disseminated to all the primary health care centres and are available in hard copy (paper form). Since existing guidelines have only recently been developed they have not yet been formally audited, but plans are in progress for this to take place in the near future. More primary care guidelines are currently under development.

At the national level no guidelines exist on the prevention and treatment of type 2 diabetes mellitus in Malta. Three clinical guidelines are currently in place at Mater Dei Hospital for the acute management of diabetic emergencies, developed by the Department of Medicine: (i) Management of Hypoglycemia, (ii) Management of Diabetic Ketoacidosis, and (iii) Perioperative Diabetes Management.

Clinicians working at the Diabetes and Endocrine Centre at Mater Dei Hospital follow international guidelines, including those of the European Association for the Study of Diabetes (EASD), the ADA and the United Kingdom's NICE. Their service is periodically evaluated through clinical audits.

As outlined in the Strategy for the Prevention and Control of Noncommunicable Disease (Department of Health Promotion and Disease Prevention, 2010), plans exist to create national guidelines for the prevention of diabetes and to integrate them with those for the prevention of obesity, CVD and cancer. These national guidelines are to be developed by a committee, which will be formed of diabetes experts, public health experts, government representatives and representatives of patients' organizations and civil society.

Spain

Background, policy context and regulatory basis

In 2006, the Quality Agency of the Ministry of Health in Spain rolled out in 2006 a quality programme called "Clinical Practice Guideline Programme in the Spanish National Health System", coordinated by GuíaSalud. GuíaSalud is tasked with developing clinical guidelines nationally and promoting their implementation through handbooks and recommendations. It also runs a guideline national clearinghouse that includes clinical guidelines in Spanish (GuíaSalud, 2012b). In this general context, clinical guidelines – including the type 2 diabetes mellitus guideline – have been developed through collaboration agreements between the Spanish Ministry of Health (through its Quality Agency) and the HTA agencies or units from Spain's various Autonomous Communities (regions).

The diabetes guideline includes all aspects of type 2 diabetes mellitus management (such as diabetic foot care, eye screening and cardiovascular management). A National Strategy on Diabetes exists, including the implementation of guidelines and standards. However, competences in health policy have been transferred to the regional governments and the level of implementation of clinical guidelines varies a great deal across regions. Finally, primary care network of professionals specialized in diabetes (GEDAPS), has a web page that publishes guidelines and other relevant content.

As mentioned before, clinical guidelines are commissioned by the Clinical Practice Guideline Programme in the Spanish National Health System and developed by evidence-based medicine institutions, mainly HTA Agencies or units from the different Autonomous Communities and are most commonly of financial nature, through services purchase contracts.

Development and implementation

The clinical guidelines development process is commissioned by the Clinical Practice Guideline Programme in the Spanish National Health System, coordinated by GuíaSalud. It is carried out by evidence-based medicine institutions, mainly HTA agencies or units from the different Autonomous Communities. Through GuíaSalud, the Quality Agency of the Ministry of Health coordinates the process of elaboration and publication of guidelines, establishing agreements with the different agencies/units and groups of experts tasked with developing the guidelines in each case. Several clinical guidelines are promoted independently by HTA agencies or professional bodies. For example, the type 2 diabetes mellitus guideline was commissioned by the Guideline Programme and developed by the Basque Health Technology Assessment Agency (OSTEBA).

The group of professionals involved in the development of a clinical guideline can include different disciplines spanning health professionals, librarians, epidemiologists, health economists, statisticians and policy-makers, depending on the topic. In the case of type 2 diabetes mellitus, four different groups of clinicians were involved: general practitioners, endocrinologists, nurses and pharmacists. Patients have been increasingly involved in guideline development, and the most relevant patients' associations are usually consulted. The exact form of this collaboration varies across guidelines, but consensus is usually achieved through debate. In the case of type 2 diabetes mellitus, focus groups were used to capture patients' views.

Clinical guidelines operate at regional level, as the Autonomous Communities are the bodies responsible for their implementation. Tools to promote their utilization – such as IT applications – are generally rare and vary depending on the regional government concerned. For example, in Basque Country, electronic reminders related to diabetes treatment (guideline updates and follow-up guides for the treatment of chronic patients) have been implemented.

The GuíaSalud web site makes clinical guidelines available to patients and professionals and provides tools for clinician such as "quick" versions of the guideline). The National Programme publishes an implementation handbook, and some Autonomous Communities have their own specific strategies for implementation. In addition, several Autonomous Communities also have their own tools to make guidelines available to professionals (agencies/units, web pages). In Basque Country, a specific web page developed in the context of a clinical trial to assess the effectiveness of cardiovascular guidelines (diabetes, hypertension and hyperlipidaemia as a cardiovascular risk factor) is now available to all professionals.

Quality control and evaluation

Quality Control measures include the use of the AGREE tool and the advice of external reviewers. These measures are not mandatory, but are as a rule followed by the HTA agencies and units within the regions. GuíaSalud tests the quality of the clinical guidelines before including them in the Spanish official clearinghouse. In the Clinical Practice Guideline Programme it is also mandatory to follow the handbook for developing clinical guidelines (GuíaSalud, 2012c).

There is no formal evaluation at any stage of the process (development, quality control or implementation). However, the quality of the clinical guidelines has improved since the publication of the aforementioned handbook and the implementation of quality control measures such as the AGREE tool. Progress regarding the implementation and evaluation of clinical guidelines is now among the priorities of the Clinical Practice Guideline Programme.

Slovenia

Background, regulatory basis, policy and strategy

There is no national agency responsible for the development and implementation of clinical guidelines in Slovenia and no comprehensive set of guidelines. International guidelines are is used on an ad hoc basis. Many guidelines and recommendations have been published in peer review journals, including the *Slovene Medical Journal*, but these are developed by groups of experts and their development methodology is rarely stated. National guidelines and standards for type 2 diabetes mellitus were recently published in a comprehensive booklet, but its content has not been endorsed by the Health Council and its use remains voluntary.

Following the St Vincent declaration,[7] a first attempt was made to make a National Diabetes Plan (NDP), along with the development of a first national diabetes clinical guideline in 2006. Though initially unsuccessful, the NDP was approved by the government in April 2010. The first Action Plan is now successfully under way, including the fast-paced preparation of clinical guidelines for all diabetes types. The most appropriate method of clinical guideline implementation in the country has yet to be designed, particularly in terms of determining resource availability.

There is no legal framework or official basis for clinical guideline development and implementation in Slovenia. However, in 2003 the Ministry of Health published the *Manual on development of clinical practice guidelines* (Slovenian Ministry of Health, 2003). This informed the development of the first diabetes clinical guideline in 2006. In diabetology, clinical guidelines have thus been based on the definition of the Ministry of Health, and best possible practice based on the best available evidence.

Development and implementation

The diabetes GDG included mainly diabetologists, but also interventional and non-interventional cardiologists; ophthalmologists; neurologists; specialists in infectious disease, hypertension and periodontal disease; gynaecologists; representatives of family physicians; and registered nurses with special knowledge in the field of diabetes. Patients were not included in the development of the guidelines; however, a special version targeted towards patients is being prepared. It is envisaged that a patient representative will actively participate in the next update. Consensus within the working group was based mostly on available evidence supplemented by expert opinion (see Chapter 6 for more information on guideline development in general in Slovenia).

The use of guidelines is not mandatory in Slovenia. They are generally poorly implemented and their implementation is inadequately assessed. However, a pocket version of the diabetes guidelines has been distributed to all family physicians; diabetologists; registered nurses with special knowledge in the diabetes field; every hospital with an internal medicine department; relevant resident physicians; all members of the coordinating group of the NDP; representatives of the Ministry of Health and the Health Insurance Institute; and patient representatives. This publication is also available at every conference or meeting related to diabetes and organized by stakeholders involved in clinical guideline development. Moreover, an online version has been developed and can be freely accessed by everybody of interest.

---

7 The St Vincent Declaration includes a set of goals for the medical care of people with diabetes mellitus, published in 1989.

Other tools that have been considered for quality improvement include clinical pathways as a coordination aid for diabetes, to be developed along with the NDP. The possibility of developing Disease Management Programmes has recently been discussed, and primary care model practices have been piloted in 2011, in terms of restructuring the delivery of care (nurse-led care coordination). In addition, decision algorithms for diabetes are being developed.

Quality control and evaluation

Clinical guidelines are not checked for quality before being implemented. For diabetes guidance, no standardized tool was used in guideline development and the evidence was graded according to the ADA tool, adapted for the Slovenian context. Although the AGREE tool itself was not used for quality control when developing the diabetes guideline, many of the aspects of the AGREE instrument have been incorporated in the process. The approach of using limited resource availability was not addressed directly and the perspective of thinking of the individual patient prevails. Certain chapters of the guidelines identify organizational, financial and other resource barriers as being considerable. In addition, the issue of conflicts of interest is not explicitly dealt with.

The development, quality control, implementation and use of the diabetes guidelines have not been evaluated so far.

Conclusions

Type 2 diabetes mellitus is a highly prevalent, multifaceted chronic condition in Europe, and one for which there are well-established prevention, treatment and management initiatives in most European countries. Thus, type 2 diabetes mellitus was an interesting window through which to understand the status of clinical guideline production in different contexts, because even countries in which clinical guidelines are in their infancy are likely to have tackled this condition to some extent.

The case of type 2 diabetes mellitus clearly illustrates the cooperation between coordinating bodies and specialist professional associations within guideline production. For example, in Germany, the expertise of the DDG is clearly sought to assist guideline production, both in general and specifically for the Disease Management Programmes, for which decisions are made by the G-BA. Furthermore, the case studies also clearly illustrate the two-way practice of national guidelines adapted at the local level and local guidelines informing national recommendations (England and Spain respectively).

Type 2 diabetes mellitus guidance reflects the general situation regarding stakeholder involvement: countries with many years of experience in clinical guideline production have established standards for stakeholder involvement, most importantly the inclusion of patients via patient associations (England, France and Germany). In other cases, where such mechanisms are still lacking, patient involvement is recognized as a goal for the future (Slovenia).

The multidisciplinarity of GDGs is a common characteristic of almost all case studies, reflecting the recognition of the need for a comprehensive approach for chronic conditions such as diabetes.

It is interesting to see that in countries with long-established clinical guideline production systems, such as England and Germany, several pieces of guidance are produced for the same condition, encompassing as many aspects of care as possible. The availability and dissemination of these guidelines naturally depends on the system in place: in England, the NICE integrates them in its general type 2 diabetes mellitus guidance, whereas in Germany they are individually identifiable and/or separate modules of the NVL programme.

A very important insight gained from the case studies is the utilization on behalf of health professionals of international guidelines when initiatives within the country are limited. Knowledge transfer between countries – going beyond the ad hoc use of international guidelines when context-specific information is lacking – could provide important foundations for informing less formalized processes. However, the different models of health service delivery should be taken into account before best practice material can be deemed to be transferrable. This is particularly important for conditions such as type 2 diabetes mellitus, which are treated and managed at many levels. Awareness and utilization of existing research on guideline implementation strategies for type 2 diabetes mellitus can aid developers and guidance issuers in better disseminating and evaluating their work and thus further endorsing quality of care.

Part 4

Are guidelines in Europe well developed? Are they well implemented? Do they have any impact? A systematic review of the literature

S Brusamento, C Knai, H Legido-Quigley, D Panteli, E Turk, V Saliba, J Car, M McKee and R Busse

Introduction

The previous sections of this report have mapped out the development and implementation of clinical guidelines in the EU and have described the development and implementation of a guideline for managing a specific chronic disease (adult type 2 diabetes mellitus). However, while it has been possible to provide a detailed account of what is happening in Europe, the descriptions in this report were not able to capture whether clinical guidelines were of good quality or met the AGREE criteria; whether the strategies to disseminate and implement clinical guidelines were appropriate; and whether these had an impact on medical practice. The following sections aim to fill in this gap by systematically searching the literature in these three broad areas. Therefore, this section addresses three different questions, and is based on three literature searches, in each case focusing on reviews and studies from European countries. It is hoped that this will provide policy-makers with additional information about the evidence available on the development, dissemination and implementation – as well as impact – of clinical guidelines in the European context. A lack of evidence does not necessarily mean that clinical guidelines are not effective. In order to follow the discussion on how best to coordinate clinical guidelines, two complementary approaches are needed: (i) to provide a description of what is currently happening across Europe (mapping exercise) and (ii) to present the evidence available on how well carried out and effective these initiatives are (systematic reviews).

Objectives

The specific objectives of this systematic review are:

- to assess whether clinical guidelines that have been developed in EU countries are of high quality (as to whether they meet the AGREE criteria);

- to identify the most effective strategies to disseminate and implement clinical guidelines in EU countries;

- to evaluate the impact of the use of clinical guidelines on medical practice (processes) and patient outcomes.

Methods

Search and screening

Three databases (CENTRAL, MEDLINE and EMBASE) were searched, applying the general search strategy that is presented in Annex 3 (Table A3.1). Only studies published since the year 2000 and performed in EU countries were considered. Included studies were required to focus on the following selected chronic conditions in adults: coronary heart disease, COPD, asthma, type 2 diabetes mellitus, arthritis (defined broadly to include all types of chronic arthritis conditions, such as osteoarthritis as well as rheumatoid arthritis), breast cancer, cervical cancer, colorectal cancer, and depressive disorder.

The search results were merged in a single database and duplicates removed. Subsequently, citations were screened against inclusion criteria. Different inclusion criteria were applied during this process to select studies which met the criteria for the three objectives of this review: (i) development of clinical guidelines; (ii) dissemination and implementation of clinical guidelines; and (iii) impact of clinical guidelines (Table 4.1).

Table 4.1 *Selection criteria for included studies according to the three main objectives*

Development	Dissemination and implementation	Impact
	Aim	
To evaluate the quality of clinical guidelines developed in EU countries, for the management of the included conditions according to the AGREE criteria.	To assess the effectiveness of different strategies to disseminate and implement clinical guidelines.	To assess the impact of using clinical guidelines in medical practice.
	Study design	
Evaluation studies of clinical guidelines were included. [Due to the topic, neither interventional nor observational studies were considered.]	High-quality rigorous evaluations were considered: RCT, c-RCT, CCT, CBA and ITS.	High-quality rigorous evaluations were considered: RCT, c-RCT, CCT, CBA and ITS. To allow the assessment of the effectiveness of clinical guidelines during routine practice, observational studies and cross-sectional surveys were also considered that assessed the desired outcomes before and after the introduction of clinical guidelines.
	Participants	
No limitations	Health care professionals	Health care professionals and patients

Table 4.1 *contd*

Development	Dissemination and implementation	Impact
	Intervention	
Studies were included if they appraised clinical guidelines using the AGREE instrument.	Studies were required to assess the dissemination and/or implementation of clinical guidelines for the care of the previously cited chronic conditions. Studies could compare one or more interventions to a control group, or two or more interventions with each other without having a control group. The implementation strategy could involve a single intervention as well as multifaceted interventions. The intervention had to involve the active participation of health care professional(s); e.g., studies on the use of automated reminders sent to patients to remind them to attend an appointment were not included; nor were studies that determine the feasibility and effectiveness of using specific devices (e.g. portable spirometer, electronical record system).	Studies had to assess the impact of clinical guidelines on the management of the previously cited chronic conditions. Studies could compare two groups, one applying the clinical guidelines and the second not applying them, regardless of the methods used to implement them. Studies that compared two different implementation strategies with no control group were not considered for this topic. Studies could also measure the outcome before and after the dissemination or implementation of the clinical guidelines.
	Outcome	
The methodological quality of clinical guidelines had to be assessed using quantitative objective data, such as scores reporting the quality of various criteria (e.g. the AGREE quality domains).	The effectiveness of the intervention had to be measured by using quantitative objective data, such as performance indicators reporting on process of care, prescription, and patients' health outcomes. Studies only reporting on physician knowledge or those that presented self-reported outcome (collected by questioning either health care professionals or patients) were not considered.	In order to reduce overlap with the implementation chapter, high-quality, rigorous evaluations were included only if they reported on patients' health impact. Other study designs were also included if they reported either on process of care or patients' health impact. Only studies reporting quantitative objective data on the above indicators were considered. Studies that reported on patients' satisfaction and/or self-reported outcomes were not considered.

Data extraction and analysis

Relevant data were extracted from all the included studies using a standardized form. The information extracted for the three sections of this review is presented in Annex 3 (Table A3.2). Since the outcome measurement varied across the recommendations, it was not possible to pool the results of different studies and provide an estimate of effectiveness. Therefore, a narrative synthesis was conducted to report the results for the three topics.

In order to present the effectiveness of implementation and health impact of clinical guidelines, it was necessary to summarize the results of studies having rigorous study design using the same strategy that Lugtenberg et al. adopted (Lugtenberg, Burgers & Westert, 2009). Thus, the assessment of effectiveness was allocated to three categories: mostly effective ("++"), if there was a significant effect on more than 50% of the indicators; partly effective ("+"), if there was significant effect on 50% or less of the indicators; and not effective when no significant effect was demonstrated for any of the indicators.

Studies that assessed the effectiveness of guideline implementation versus no intervention and reported on patients' health outcome were considered twice – first, for the evaluation of implementation strategies and second, for their impact if they met the inclusion criteria.

Results

Result of the literature search

The search strategy yielded 853 citations (see Annex 3, Table A3.3 and Table A3.4). After removing duplicates and screening, four studies met the inclusion criteria for the evaluation of guidelines quality, 10 studies for the assessment of implementation (Frijling et al., 2002; Van Bruggen et al., 2008; Verstappen et al., 2003; Asmar, 2007; Baker et al., 2003; Hormigo Pozo et al., 2009; Lagerlov et al., 2000b; Perria et al., 2007; Rosemann et al., 2007; Sondergaard et al., 2002) and six for the assessment of impact (Lub et al., 2006; Van Bruggen et al., 2008; Asmar, 2007; Rosemann et al., 2007; Smith et al., 2008; Tinelli et al., 2003). Three of the studies included in the assessment of implementation were also included in the impact assessments (Van Bruggen et al., 2008; Asmar, 2007; Rosemann et al., 2007). The reasons for exclusion of studies after the full text analysis are reported in Annex 3 (Table A3.5, Table A3.6 and Table A3.7). The selection process is shown in Fig. 4.1 using an adapted PRISMA approach (Preferred Reporting Items for Systematic Reviews and Meta-Analyses).

Fig. 4.1 *PRISMA[a] flow diagram*

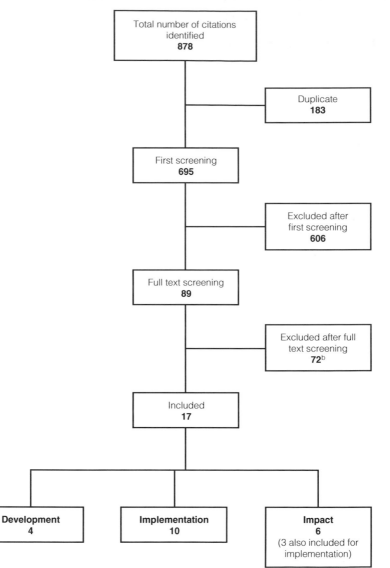

[a] See the PRISMA Statement for further details (BMJ, 2009); [b] See reasons for exclusions in Annex 3, Table A3.5, A3.6 and A3.7.

The studies were undertaken in only 10 out of the 27 EU countries. One study reported on the effectiveness of implementation strategies of clinical guidelines for asthma (Lagerlov et al., 2000b) – it formed part of a multicentre qualitative study (on attitudes of general practitioners in Germany, the Netherlands, Norway, Slovakia and Sweden (Lagerlov et al., 2000a); although the part of the study that reported on effectiveness of implementation was only performed in Norway, and this study was included).

The national distribution is presented in Fig. 4.2; where studies assessed clinical guidelines in more than one country, each is counted separately.

Fig. 4.2 *Distribution of included studies by country (10 EU countries plus Norway)*

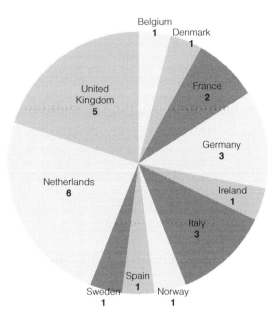

The search sought out studies related to nine chronic conditions; however, studies that met inclusion criteria only addressed seven of those conditions, as shown in Fig. 4.3. Studies were counted more than once if they included multiple conditions.

Fig. 4.3 *Distribution of number of studies for each chronic condition*

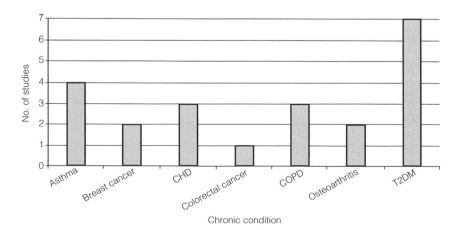

Methodological quality of clinical guidelines

Description of studies

Four studies were included analysing a total of 21 European guidelines. Two studies focused on cancers (breast (Wennekes et al., 2008) and colorectal (Watine & Bunting, 2008)), and two on type 2 diabetes mellitus (Stone et al., 2010; Nagy et al., 2008).

The countries in which the analysed guidelines were developed were: Belgium (1), France (1), Germany (3), Ireland (1), Italy (1), Netherlands (3), United Kingdom (10, of which England (1), Scotland (2), Wales (1), and the United Kingdom (6)). The scope of the guidelines varied: two studies analysed guidelines dealing with the diagnosis, treatment and/or management of type 2 diabetes mellitus (Stone et al., 2010; Nagy et al., 2008), one on the screening and/or treatment of breast cancer (Wennekes et al., 2008), and one on the diagnosis and/or treatment of colorectal cancer (Watine & Bunting, 2008).

All four studies appraised clinical guidelines using the AGREE instrument and reported their results according to the AGREE quality domain scores.

Guidelines quality scores

All four of the studies reported results in terms of scores for each AGREE domain. The study characteristics, individual and mean scores, and appraisers' final recommendations are reported in Table 4.2.

There was considerable variation in the quality of clinical guidelines according to the AGREE instrument domains. The mean "Scope and purpose" (D1 in Table 4.2) score was 86%, ranging from 33% to 100%. This domain was the most adequately addressed, with scores above 80% in 17 out of 21 clinical guidelines. It was followed by the "Clarity of presentation" (D4) domain, with a mean score of 83%, ranging from 54% to 100%, and with scores above 80% in 14 out of 21 clinical guidelines.

The "Stakeholder involvement" (D2 in Table 4.2) domain was less addressed, and only four out of 21 clinical guidelines scored above 80%. This domain had a mean score of 61%, ranging from 8% to 88%. The clinical guidelines performed similarly in the "Rigour of development" (D3) domain, with a mean score of 69%, ranging from 31% to 95%. Only six out of 21 clinical guidelines scored above 80%.

The last two domains were the least well-tackled. The mean "Applicability" score (D5 in Table 4.2) was 46%, ranging from 6% to 100%, with only two clinical guidelines scoring above 80%, and 12 clinical guidelines out of 21 scored 50% or less. The mean "Editorial Independence" score (D6) was 48%,

Table 4.2 *Characteristics and AGREE domain score (%) for European guidelines analysed and reported in four studies*

Studies	Country/Year of publication	Clinical subject	Institution	Type of institution	AGREE domain score (%)[a]						Appraisers' recommendations
					D1	D2	D3	D4	D5	D6	
Nagy et al., 2008	United Kingdom (Scotland) 2001	Type 2 Diabetes Mellitus	SIGN	Governmental	56	75	74	71	8	71	Strongly recommend
	United Kingdom 2002	Type 2 Diabetes Mellitus	NICE	Governmental	92	85	87	98	33	42	Strongly recommend
	United Kingdom 2002	Type 2 Diabetes Mellitus	NICE	Governmental	92	88	90	98	33	42	Strongly recommend
	United Kingdom 2004	Type 2 Diabetes Mellitus	NCCWCH (NICE)	Governmental	97	88	92	98	72	92	Strongly recommend
	United Kingdom 2007	Type 2 Diabetes Mellitus	NHS/CKS	Governmental	97	71	64	90	56	21	Strongly recommend
	United Kingdom 2007	Type 2 Diabetes Mellitus	NHS/CKS	Governmental	97	69	67	88	56	21	Strongly recommend
	United Kingdom 2007	Type 2 Diabetes Mellitus	NHS/CKS	Governmental	75	71	67	81	72	29	Strongly recommend
Stone et al., 2010	Belgium 2005	Type 2 Diabetes Mellitus	FAGP/FDA	Medical society	89	83	88	79	50	100	Recommend with provisos or alterations
	United Kingdom (England and Wales) 2008	Type 2 Diabetes Mellitus	NCCCC	Governmental	100	75	95	100	100	100	Strongly recommended
	France 2006	Type 2 Diabetes Mellitus	HAS	Governmental	33	8	76	92	6	17	Recommend with provisos or alterations
	Germany 2002	Type 2 Diabetes Mellitus	GCC	Governmental	83	29	64	58	17	50	Recommend with provisos or alterations
	Ireland 2008	Type 2 Diabetes Mellitus	HSE	Governmental	83	21	48	96	33	0	Recommend with provisos or alterations

Table 4.2 contd

Studies	Country/Year of publication	Clinical subject	Institution	Type of institution	AGREE domain score (%)[a]						Appraisers' recommendations
					D1	D2	D3	D4	D5	D6	
Stone et al., 2010	Italy 2007	Type 2 Diabetes Mellitus	IAD/ISD	Medical society	61	58	60	83	44	0	Recommend with provisos or alterations
	Netherlands 2006	Type 2 Diabetes Mellitus	NHG	Medical society	100	71	31	96	72	83	Strongly recommended
	Sweden 2000	Type 2 Diabetes Mellitus	SMPA	Governmental	100	46	71	75	89	83	Strongly recommended
Watine & Bunting, 2008	United Kingdom 2000	Colorectal cancer	BSG/RCP/ACGBI	Medical society	89	21	33	54	67	0	Would not recommend
	United Kingdom (Scotland) 2003	Colorectal cancer	SIGN	Governmental	100	58	57	67	6	0	Would not recommend
Wennekes et al., 2008	Netherlands 2000	Breast cancer	CBO	Governmental	83	69	52	73	25	29	*Not reported*
	Netherlands 2004	Breast cancer	CBO	Governmental	97	73	65	83	14	46	*Not reported*
	Germany 2003	Breast cancer	German Society for Senology	Medical society	89	71	75	81	72	88	*Not reported*
	Germany 2004	Breast cancer	AWMF	Governmental	100	54	89	90	42	96	*Not reported*
Mean domain scores					**86**	**61**	**69**	**83**	**46**	**48**	

[a] AGREE domain scores: D1: scope and purpose; D2: stakeholder involvement; D3: rigour of development; D4: clarity of presentation; D5: applicability; D6: editorial independence.

ranging from 0% to 100%: seven out of 21 clinical guidelines scored above 80%, but the majority scored 50% or less, including four which scored 0%, making the "Editorial independence" domain the least well-completed.

Nagy et al. (2008), Stone et al. (2010) and Watine & Bunting (2008) (between them analysing 17 European guidelines) included an overall assessment: 10 out of 17 were "strongly recommended", five out of 17 were recommended with provisos or alterations, and two out of 17 were not recommended. Five clinical guidelines were developed by medical societies and 16 by governmental institutions; there was no marked difference in quality scores.

Several studies on the quality of European clinical guidelines were just outside the scope of this review but contribute important insights. A description is included here for that reason.

Voellinger et al. (2003) analysed the quality of guidelines for the management of **depressive disorders** using the AGREE instrument, but reported limited results. They reported that there was a lack of high-quality evidence in the existing recommendations for the management of depressive disorders: of the six European guidelines analysed, three did not present any evidence for their clinical recommendations. However, they included guidelines developed between 1997 and 2001, which is before the development of the AGREE criteria.

Delgado-Noguera et al. (2009) analysed the quality of 22 clinical practice guidelines for the **prevention and treatment of childhood overweight and obesity**, using the AGREE method. They also reported poor involvement of stakeholders in the process of guideline development (with a mean score of 34%), modest results for rigour of development (with a mean score of 35%) and low results for applicability (24.5%). They concluded that only half of the 22 clinical guidelines on the prevention and treatment of overweight and obesity in childhood published between 1998 and 2007 were evidence based, and that only six could be recommended and applied. They warned that lack of rigorous evaluation of the best available evidence could lead to unreliable and harmful recommendations for patients.

Smith et al. (2003) assessed the quality of COPD guidelines, according to eight quality criteria (applicability, validity, reproducibility, clinical flexibility, clarity, multidisciplinarity, documentation, and scheduled review) set out by Ward & Grieco (1996). Two of the seven guidelines reviewed were European, developed by the European Respiratory Society (1995) and the British Thoracic Society (BTS) (1997) respectively. They found that validity of the development processes of published guidelines was limited. Moreover, consumer participation was not reported for any of the reviewed guidelines, except for contributions from a lay group in the development of the BTS guideline.

Gaebel et al. (2005) analysed 14 European practice guidelines on the management and treatment of **schizophrenia**, published between 1994 and 2004, using the AGREE instrument. They found the methodological quality of many schizophrenia guidelines to be "modest" at best. Stakeholder involvement was poorly addressed in most guidelines (three out of 14 scored 0% in the "stakeholder involvement" domain, and all but one guideline scored less than 42%); few guidelines consulted stakeholders other than psychiatrists in their development process. The authors also found the guidelines to be poorly applicable (seven out of 14 scored 0% on the "applicability" domain).

Effects of implementation strategies

Description of studies

Ten studies were included, all of which were developed in primary care and involved general practitioners. The studies' characteristics are presented in Annex 3 (Table A3.8).

One study each was performed in Denmark (Sondergaard et al., 2002), France (Asmar, 2007), Germany (Rosemann et al., 2007), Italy (Perria et al., 2007), Norway (Lagerlov et al., 2000b), Spain (Hormigo Pozo et al., 2009) and the United Kingdom (Baker et al., 2003), and three studies were carried out in the Netherlands (Frijling et al., 2002; Van Bruggen et al., 2008; Verstappen et al., 2003).

One was a controlled before-and-after (CBA) study (Hormigo Pozo et al., 2009), two studies were randomized controlled trials (RCTs) (Asmar, 2007; Sondergaard et al., 2002), and the other seven studies were cluster-randomized controlled trials (c-RCTs), for which the randomization process occurred at practice level.

Four studies focused on guidelines for management and care of type 2 diabetes mellitus (Frijling et al., 2002; Van Bruggen et al., 2008; Hormigo Pozo et al., 2009; Perria et al., 2007), one study on osteoarthritis management (Rosemann et al., 2007), one on hypertension (Asmar, 2007), two on asthma (Lagerlov et al., 2000b; Sondergaard et al., 2002), one on asthma and coronary heart disease (Baker et al., 2003), and two evaluated guidelines for COPD, asthma, coronary heart disease and degenerative arthritis (Verstappen et al., 2003; Baker et al., 2003).

Five studies implemented national guidelines (Frijling et al., 2002; Van Bruggen et al., 2008; Verstappen et al., 2003; Baker et al., 2003; Sondergaard et al., 2002), one study implemented European guidelines (Asmar, 2007) and four studies adapted international guidelines to the context of a specific country (Hormigo Pozo et al., 2009; Lagerlov et al., 2000b; Perria et al., 2007; Rosemann et al., 2007).

The distribution of studies by the country of implementation and chronic condition focused on is presented in Fig. 4.4. Each condition that a study focused on was counted separately, thus a study was able to contribute to more than one condition.

Fig. 4.4 *Distribution studies by country of implementation, chronic condition and type of guidelines (national or not)*

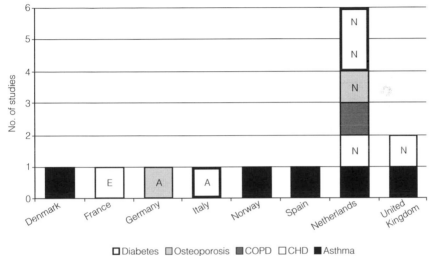

☐Diabetes ▨Osteoporosis ■COPD ☐CHD ■Asthma

Notes: Guidelines: N: national, E: European; A: adapted from international.

Effectiveness of implementation strategies

Single intervention versus control

Three studies implemented a single intervention compared to no intervention (control group) (Van Bruggen et al., 2008; Perria et al., 2007; Sondergaard et al., 2002), of which two were ineffective, while one study was partially effective.

Two studies focused on guidelines for type 2 diabetes mellitus, both of which were c-RCTs. The first implemented national clinical guidelines using educational outreach visits (Van Bruggen et al., 2008), while the second assessed the effectiveness of two single interventions, namely, formal training of general practitioners and a mail dissemination of clinical guidelines, versus no intervention (Perria et al., 2007). The third study was an RCT assessing the effectiveness of two different kinds of feedback relating to national guidelines on prescribing for asthma, versus no intervention. One group of general practitioners received detailed feedback showing the number of patients that they treated categorized by kind of drugs prescribed and dosage; no comparison with other practices was provided. The second group received aggregated data whereby all the practices were categorized according to the total number of prescriptions per 100 patients they produced, regardless of the specific drug and dosage (Sondergaard et al., 2002).

Only the use of educational outreach visits (Van Bruggen et al., 2008) led to significant improvement in the process of care (fasting blood glucose measurement, blood pressure control, body weight control, $p<0.01$ after adjustment for covariates) but it did not translate into any significant difference in health outcomes.

Multifaceted intervention

The other seven studies assessed multifaceted interventions. Six studies compared multifaceted interventions to no intervention, while one compared two single interventions versus a multifaceted intervention (Baker et al., 2003). One of those studies showed no effect (Baker et al., 2003), four studies were "partly" effective (Frijling et al., 2002; Verstappen et al., 2003; Lagerlov et al., 2000b; Rosemann et al., 2007), and two studies were "mostly" effective (Asmar, 2007; Hormigo Pozo et al., 2009), even though one of the latter had a poor design.

The individual interventions applied in the studies included are summarized in Table 4.3.

Table 4.3 *Interventions used in multifaceted implementation strategies*

Intervention	Number of studies
Educational outreach visits	2
Formal training	1
Small educational meetings	5
Educational material for general practitioners	5
Educational material for patients' education	1
Feedback to general practitioners	5

Six different combinations of interventions were evaluated (Table 4.4): two c-RCTs employed two interventions (Baker et al., 2003; Rosemann et al., 2007); three c-RCTs and one RCT combined three strategies (Frijling et al., 2002; Verstappen et al., 2003; Asmar, 2007; Lagerlov et al., 2000b); and one CBA study used four interventions (Hormigo Pozo et al., 2009). Since the combinations that were implemented differed for each study, it was not possible to pool their results to obtain an estimate of the effectiveness of each combination.

Table 4.4 *Combinations of multifaceted implementations*

Combinations of interventions	Number of studies (relevant reference)
Educational outreach visits + Educational material for general practitioners + Feedback	1 (Frijling et al., 2002)
Educational outreach visits + Educational material for general practitioners + Workshops	1 (Asmar, 2007)
Feedback + Workshops + Educational material for general practitioners + Formal training	1 (Hormigo Pozo et al., 2009)
Feedback + Workshops + Educational material for general practitioners	2 (Verstappen et al., 2003; Lagerlov et al., 2000b)
Feedback + Educational material for general practitioners	1 (Baker et al., 2003)
Workshops + Educational material for patients	1 (Rosemann et al., 2007)

Multifaceted interventions incorporating educational outreach visits

Each of the studies using educational outreach visits resulted in significant improvement of some of the assessed outcomes. The one on type 2 diabetes mellitus guidelines showed partial effectiveness: two out of the seven measured processes of care significantly improved (Odds ratio (OR) for foot examination 1.68, 95%CI 1.19–2.39; OR for eye examination 1.52, 95%CI 1.07–2.16); however, there was no improvement in prescribing (Frijling et al., 2002). The second study was "mostly effective", although it only had one outcome. The study focused on hypertension guidelines; significantly more patients achieved blood pressure control in the intervention group (47.8% versus 44.7%, p=0.005), although the prescribing pattern was similar in the intervention and the control groups (Asmar, 2007).

Multifaceted interventions incorporating feedback

Five studies combined feedback on performance to general practitioners with other interventions (Frijling et al., 2002; Verstappen et al., 2003; Baker et al., 2003; Hormigo Pozo et al., 2009; Lagerlov et al., 2000b); one was effective (Hormigo Pozo et al., 2009), three showed partial effectiveness (Frijling et al., 2002; Verstappen et al., 2003; Lagerlov et al., 2000b) and one showed no effect (Baker et al., 2003).

In two studies the general practitioner received individualized feedback on their performance during the duration of the study (Frijling et al., 2002; Hormigo Pozo et al., 2009). In two other studies the general practitioners received individualized feedback on process of care and prescriptions, but only during the workshops used to disseminate the clinical guidelines; in both of these studies, participants also received educational material (Verstappen et al.,

2003; Lagerlov et al., 2000b). Finally, in one study the general practitioner received only one instance of feedback on their practice performance (Baker et al., 2003).

All four studies that combined personalized feedback with two or more other interventions showed some effectiveness, even if the results were heterogeneous, while the study providing feedback at practice level did not show any effectiveness. The studies providing continuous feedback had slightly better results compared to the others.

The two studies which provided continuous feedback during the intervention focused on the type 2 diabetes mellitus guideline. In one study, two out of seven process of care indicators improved (Frijling et al., 2002). In the second, both process of care (Relative Risk 9.74 for cardiovascular risk assessment, after the intervention between the two groups, p=0.0001) and prescribing behaviour (relative risk 1.407, p<0.05) were significantly better after the intervention. However, the analysis of the latter (a CBA study) was weak, mostly focusing on the comparison of two groups (intervention versus no intervention) after the implementation (Hormigo Pozo et al., 2009).

The two studies which provided individualized feedback only during the training phase combined that feedback with a workshop and the provision of educational material. In the study comparing asthma guidelines implementation versus no intervention, the proportion of patients treated according to the guidelines significantly improved in the intervention group (relative increase 5.9% (variance 2.5), p=0.018) (Lagerlov et al., 2000b). The second study compared two intervention groups with each other: one implementing guidelines on coronary heart disease and hypertension and the other implementing guidelines on COPD and asthma. Each group acted as control for the other. The study resulted in an improvement of the primary outcome (decrease in the total numbers of requested tests: intervention effect ß –35, (95%CI –61 to –10), p=0.01) only for coronary heart diseases, while there was no difference in the asthma group. Moreover, there was no difference in the number of inappropriate tests requested in either of the groups (Verstappen et al., 2003).

Finally, one c-RCT compared three different ways to disseminate clinical guidelines: two single interventions and a multifaceted intervention. One group of general practitioners received the full version of two guidelines (for asthma and for angina; 51 and 59 recommendations, respectively); the second group received a short version containing only the strongest recommendations (10 and 14, respectively); and the third group received the short version plus a single instance of feedback on practice performance. None of the strategies was significantly more effective than any of the others (Baker et al., 2003).

Multifaceted interventions incorporating educational material

All the studies which applied multifaceted interventions containing either outreach visits or feedback were associated with the provision of educational material to the general practitioners.

Moreover, a study on the implementation of osteoarthritis management guidelines associated the provision of training for general practitioners with the use of educational material for physicians and patients. The control group received no intervention. The intervention did not affect the patients' utilization of health services or quality of life. The only significant improvement was in the percentage of prescriptions of acetaminophen (p<0.001) (Rosemann et al., 2007).

Impact of clinical guidelines on process of care and patients' health outcomes

Description of studies

Six studies were included, all evaluating the impact of clinical guidelines in primary care. The characteristics of the studies included are displayed in Table 4.5.

Two were performed in the Netherlands (Lub et al., 2006; Van Bruggen et al., 2008) and one each in France (Asmar, 2007), Germany (Rosemann et al., 2007), Italy (Tinelli et al., 2003) and the United Kingdom (Smith et al., 2008).

Four had a rigorous study design, meaning that their conclusions would have low risk of bias. Three of these – one RCT (Asmar, 2007) and two c-RCTs (Van Bruggen et al., 2008; Rosemann et al., 2007) – evaluated the effectiveness of different strategies to implement clinical guidelines and they all reported on health outcomes associated with the intervention.

The guidelines focused on were: a European guideline on management of hypertension (Asmar, 2007), a national guideline on type 2 diabetes mellitus (Van Bruggen et al., 2008) and a European guideline (European League Against Rheumatism (EULAR)) on osteoarthritis that had been adapted for the German context (Rosemann et al., 2007). A third c-RCT randomized physicians to apply a version of a COPD guideline from the European Respiratory Society and American Thoracic Society guidelines adapted for being in an Italian region (Tinelli et al., 2003).

Table 4.5 *Characteristics of included studies for health impact evaluation*

Referencing details	Country Study design Year of study	Conditions	Guidelines	Participants	Outcome	Result	Effect size
Asmar, 2007	France RCT 2004–2005	Hypertension	European Society of Hypertension – International Society of Hypertension guidelines (2003)	Intervention: 502 physicians, 2 128 patients Control: 595 physicians, 2 308 patients	Health impact: % of patients strictly controlled according to the target level	Significant improvement (intervention 47.8% versus 44.7% (P= .005).	++
Rosemann et al., 2007	Germany c-RCT 2005	Osteoarthritis	Adapted from European guidelines (EULAR) 2001	Intervention: 25 general practitioners, 345 patients Control: 25 general practitioners, 332 patients	Health impact: quality of life	Health impact: no difference	–
Van Bruggen et al., 2008	Netherlands c-RCT Not stated	Type 2 diabetes mellitus	Locally adapted from the Practice guideline type 2 diabetes mellitus of the NHG (1999)	Intervention: 15 general practices, 822 patients Control: 15 general practices, 818 patients	Health impact: % of patients with poor glycaemic control at baseline that achieved control Mean HbA1c% value Total cholesterol value Blood pressure values Quality of life	No difference except in terms of cholesterol: small, statistically significant improvement	+
Tinelli et al., 2003	Italy c-RCT 1998–1999	COPD	Developed by a national scientific committee, adapted from the European Respiratory Society and American Thoracic Society guidelines (1995).	Intervention: 12 general practitioners, 72 patients Control: 10 general practitioners, 51 patients	Health impact: no. of episodes of exacerbations No. of hospital admissions due to COPD	No difference	–

| Lub et al., 2006 | Netherlands Cross-sectional study 1999 and 2003 | Type 2 diabetes mellitus | National practice guidelines of the NHG (1999) | Data from 53 community pharmacies, total population 450 000 people | Process of care: % of initial patients treated with the appropriate drug (patients with BMI >27 should be treated with metformin) | % of metformin as initial treatment rose from 13.4% in 1998 to 49.9% in 2003 (P= < 0.001). | N/A |
| Smith et al., 2008 | United Kingdom Cross-sectional study 2003 and 2005 | COPD | NICE Guideline for the management of COPD (February 2004) | 2003: 2 020 424 people of whom 25 565 with COPD 2005: 2 063 130 people of whom 29 870 with COPD | Process of care: recorded spirometry, drugs prescription | Recording of spirometry data executed in 18% versus 62% Prescription of combination inhaler 25% versus 44% | N/A |

Notes: Effect sizes: "++": mostly effective – there was a significant effect on more than 50% of the indicators; "+": partly effective – there was significant effect on 50% or less of the indicators; "–": not effective, no significant effect was demonstrated for any of the indicators.

In addition, two studies were included, presenting the results of cross-sectional surveys executed before and after the introduction of national guidelines for type 2 diabetes mellitus (Lub et al., 2006) and COPD (Smith et al., 2008).

Results from RCTs assessing impact on patients' health

All the studies compared the use of guidelines versus no intervention or "usual care". Only one out of the four studies showed a significant improvement in patients' health status ("mostly effective"). This was an RCT on hypertension guidelines which enrolled 502 general practitioners and their 2128 patients with hypertension in the intervention group and 595 general practitioners and their 2308 patients in the control group (usual care). The study lasted only eight weeks. The proportion of patients that achieved strict blood pressure control at the end of the study (according to the guideline target) was significantly higher in the intervention group (47.8% versus 44.7%, p=0.005) (Asmar, 2007).

The study assessing the health impact of the type 2 diabetes mellitus guideline did not show any improvement in the primary outcome (percentage of patients with poor glycaemic control at baseline achieving good control at the end: 70.4% versus 57.6%, p<0.2 after adjustment for baseline values and confounders). Only one of the secondary outcomes, total cholesterol value, significantly improved, even if only slightly (5.1±1.0 vs 5.2±1.0 mmol/l, p<0.05) (Van Bruggen et al., 2008).

The c-RCTs evaluating the patients' quality of life after the implementation of osteoarthritis management guidelines in primary care (Rosemann et al., 2007) and the study evaluating the impact of COPD guidelines (Tinelli et al., 2003) did not show any significant improvement in patients' outcomes.

Results from observational and cross-sectional studies on process of care and patients' health

One cross-sectional survey evaluated the difference in process of care, while the second assessed process of care and health impact.

The first study reviewed the initial treatment for patients with type 2 diabetes mellitus before and after the dissemination of the guidelines revised in 1999; these guideline promoted the use of a different drug for overweight/obese patients (body mass index (BMI) >27). It was found that the proportion of patients treated with the new recommended drug increased from 13.4% in 1998 to 49.9% in 2003 (p<0.001). However, the study did not measure patients' BMI, although the authors estimated that 60% of type 2 diabetes mellitus patients in that country had a BMI >27. Therefore, it cannot be asserted that the change in prescribing over time was due to adherence to the revised guidelines (Lub et al., 2006).

The second cross-sectional study aimed to evaluate the impact of the introduction of the 2004 NICE Guideline on COPD and the Quality and Outcomes Framework contract in the United Kingdom (Smith et al., 2008). Data for the years 2003 and 2005 were analysed to detect changes in process of care and whether the use of recommended treatment was associated with a reduction in mortality. The study found an improvement in the process of care (recording of spirometry data executed in 18% versus 62% of cases) and in the prescription (prescription of combination inhaler, 25% versus 44%). However, the analysis showed that in 2005 the use of the recommended treatment was associated with a higher mortality rate. This is counterintuitive. Nevertheless, the study did not take into consideration the severity of the patients' condition, so the possibility cannot be excluded that general practitioners chose to prescribe these drugs to patients with more severe disease, or the influence of some other confounders (Smith et al., 2008).

Discussion

Since the early 1990s the development and use of clinical guidelines has expanded significantly (Woolf et al., 1999). However, reliable evidence about their impact is still scarce. A systematic review of the literature on the quality of guidelines was carried out, as described, for nine conditions, analysing the effectiveness of their implementation and their health impact across the 27 EU countries. Only 17 studies were found which met the inclusion criteria: four assessing the quality of guidelines against the AGREE criteria, and 13 assessing the effectiveness of implementation or the impact of clinical guidelines. The studies included were performed in 11 different countries (10 EU countries and Norway), representing less than half of the EU countries.

Our findings are in agreement with those of Alonso-Coello et al., who conducted a systematic review of the quality of clinical guidelines developed between 1980 and 2007, across a range of clinical topics (Alonso-Coello et al., 2010). The authors reviewed 42 studies, which all used the AGREE instrument; three of those studies were included in the present report, while the other 39 studies in Alonso-Coello's review covered 605 clinical guidelines published worldwide on several different diseases. The AGREE domains – having lower scores in the present review (Stakeholder involvement, Applicability, Editorial independence) – also had lower scores in the broader review.

A previous review on the effectiveness of implementation strategies found several other evaluations, but most of them were performed in North America

(Grimshaw et al., 2004). A recent Dutch review evaluated the effectiveness of Dutch guidelines developed since the early 1990s. They used broader inclusion criteria than those used for this report. More than 200 clinical guidelines were developed in the Netherlands during the period in question; however, they found only 20 studies with an acceptable quality design and less than half assessed the health impact of guidelines. Moreover, the effect of the clinical guidelines varied largely across the studies, with a higher effect found within the studies with weaker study design and greater risk of bias in findings (Lugtenberg, Burgers & Westert, 2009). A lack of rigorous studies was also found in the analysis by Evensen et al. (2010). Within 1151 studies on clinical guidelines across nine selected conditions published between 1998 and 2007, only 28 were intervention studies with an acceptable study design and involving physicians in improving practice. Most of the others were merely descriptions of adherence, or of a process, and could not provide meaningful data on effectiveness.

Moreover, the studies focused mainly on the management of three conditions (asthma/COPD, coronary heart disease and type 2 diabetes mellitus). Although the burden of depressive disorder is high in European countries (Busse et al., 2010), only one recent paper on the evaluation of guidelines for this disorder has been found; it is the protocol of an ongoing study which should be completed at the end of 2012 (Sinnema et al., 2011). No studies were found evaluating the implementation or impact of clinical guidelines for the prevention of these three diseases.

Summary of findings: methodological quality of clinical guidelines

Four studies analysed the methodological quality of 21 European clinical guidelines focused on chronic diseases, using the AGREE appraisal instrument. The findings confirmed the conclusions of other studies; namely, that there was considerable variation in quality. This indicates a lack of consistency in relation to some aspects of the information provided to clinicians across Europe. Inconsistencies in the quality of guidelines may have an impact on the quality of recommendations made and therefore on quality of care provided to patients. Moreover, the findings consistently showed that the least well-addressed AGREE domains were usually "Stakeholder involvement", "Rigour of development", "Applicability" and "Editorial independence". This has important policy implications.

The Stakeholder involvement domain assesses the degree to which the guideline represents the views of its intended service users and providers. Recommendations should be relevant to their perceived needs. In particular it was found that consumer experiences and expectations should inform the development of the guideline; however, consumers are seldom involved in working groups and consensus groups.

The Rigour of development domain was considered particularly important by most studies, as it ensures a process of systematically reviewing the evidence on which the guidelines are developed, and an explicit link between the evidence and the recommendations. In this review only six out of 21 guidelines scored above 80% for this domain. Other studies also highlight this seeming lack of high-quality evidence in existing recommendations (Delgado-Noguera et al., 2009; Voellinger et al., 2003).

The Applicability domain evaluates issues that pertain to guideline implementation, such as organizational barriers and cost implications. Reported obstacles to guideline development include a lack of financial and human resources for developing and updating existing guidelines; and the academic approach "restricting the application of the guideline" (Gaebel et al., 2005).

The "Editorial independence" domain assesses the existence of conflicts of interest; specifically, whether the guideline was editorially independent from the funding source and from individual members of the GDG. Editorial independence was the second worst-performing domain in this review, as well as in the review conducted by Alonso-Coello et al. (2010).

Summary of findings: implementation strategies and health impact of clinical guidelines

Only two studies were "mostly effective", five studies showed partial effectiveness and three studies did not demonstrate any effectiveness. However, the results and the effect size varied across the included studies. The evaluation of the different implementation strategies showed that multifaceted implementation strategies are more effective than single interventions, and continuous feedback and outreach meetings seem to be promising strategies.

Most of the studies assessed effectiveness as being improvement in process of care. Although this is an important performance indicator, clinical guidelines aim to improve health care as a means to improving health. Only a few studies evaluated the impact on the patient and only one showed significant improvement.

The superiority of multifaceted intervention versus single intervention is consistent with the findings of previous reviews, which also found a mostly moderate effect of the different strategies of implementations (Grimshaw et al., 2004; Davis & Taylor-Vaisey, 1997).

Unfortunately, only one of the included studies presented data on the barriers to implementation of guidelines. Among the identified barriers were lack of awareness of the clinical guideline and lack of agreement with it (Van Bruggen et al., 2008). These findings are similar to those reported in a review of the barriers to guideline implementation (Cabana et al., 1999). The general assumption is that the more physicians know about guidelines, the more they will apply them. However, this assumption seems to be contradicted by the results of a recent study conducted in Germany, which showed that physicians with higher knowledge scores for selected guidelines displayed lower adherence to those same guidelines (assessed by process of care indicators) (Karbach et al., 2011).

Another common barrier to implementation mentioned by physicians is not agreeing with the recommendations (Cabana et al., 1999). Three of the 10 studies that evaluated implementation strategies included – as part of the intervention – discussion of the recommendation in small groups and/or during outreach visits; these three studies were all "mostly" (Asmar, 2007) or "partly" (Verstappen et al., 2003; Lagerlov et al., 2000b) effective.

Findings from many studies summarized by Francke et al. (2008) indicate that the simpler the guideline, the more likely that it will be accepted. However, one of the studies included – comparing the implementation of the full version of a clinical guideline versus a simple and short version – did not find significant improvement (Baker et al., 2003).

The included studies did not provide data on the cost of the dissemination or implementation of the guideline. Cost–effectiveness analysis (CEA) should include the costs of the development phase, the dissemination/implementation and the change determined in the health service by putting the guideline into practice (Vale et al., 2007). Although resources are an essential aspect of health care development, data on the cost of guideline development are scarce. A previous review including more than 200 studies on implementation strategies (only 11 from Europe) found that only 27% of them had some data on cost and only four provided data on development and implementation (one of which dated back to 1970) (Vale et al., 2007).

The strengths of the reviews in this report lie primarily in the overarching methodology, which encompasses an extensive search in numerous databases. In addition, the lack of language restrictions increased the sensitivity of the search. The fact that eventually all included studies were in English may be attributable to the tendency for robust papers to be published in international, English-language journals as well as to the sometimes limited key-wording for publications in other languages. A limitation of this study is that it was not possible to pool the results of different studies and provide an estimate of effectiveness, since outcome measures varied across recommendations.

Priorities for research

Based on the results of the review, the following research priorities can be proposed:

- to develop more rigorous studies to evaluate patients' health outcomes associated with the use of clinical guidelines;

- to assess the cost–effectiveness of developing, disseminating and implementing clinical guidelines;

- to investigate the perspective of service users and health service staff with respect to clinical guideline development and implementation (this should involve both qualitative and quantitative assessments);

- to develop more studies evaluating guidelines on prevention, depressive disorder and other mental health conditions.

Conclusions

The aim of clinical guidelines is to improve health by promoting evidence-based care. Most European countries have introduced guidelines in various forms since the early 1990s. This has involved considerable use of resources, for both developing and implementing clinical guidelines. However, the results in this report show that the evaluation of the guidelines is lacking. It is now clear that there are only a few rigorous studies assessing the quality and effectiveness of clinical guidelines in Europe. Moreover, their results are not consistent in showing a clear benefit of having clinical guidelines.

Part 5

Conclusions, policy recommendations and areas for further study

D Panteli, H Legido-Quigley, J Car, M McKee and R Busse

Clinical guidelines – as one of the tools for achieving "best practice" in health care – aim at improving health by optimizing health care provision. Available evidence on the impact of clinical guidelines on health outcomes is clearly insufficient, both in volume and robustness; a fact which is unsatisfactory, especially when taking into account the considerable resources involved in guideline production, dissemination, implementation, updating and evaluation. However, clinical guidelines have long been used in many countries as an important mechanism for quality assurance and setting standards.

Another important function of clinical guidelines is their role in synthesizing knowledge. Given the volume of clinical research published worldwide, the need for tools that bring this information together is obvious. Practitioners wishing to provide their patients with the best possible care – while spending as much time with them as possible – should have easy and comprehensive access to such information, particularly since the clinical appropriateness of the care patients are receiving largely depends on how well-informed practitioners are. However, in order for clinical guidelines to fulfil this expectation and endorse best practice while enhancing the patient–practitioner relationship, they need to be of good quality and well disseminated.

In the European context, while several countries have made impressive progress in this direction, many are still relying on sporadic and unclear processes. The level of sophistication, quality and transparency of guideline development varies substantially. The evaluation of published guidelines is the area lagging behind the most, even in well-established guidance production systems. Thus, further research and resources are required to develop more appropriate and easily implementable evaluation mechanisms, both for the appropriateness and the utilization of guidelines in place.

Even in more advanced systems, clinical guidelines focus mainly on the diagnosis and treatment of specific conditions and their complications. However, a more comprehensive approach is desirable, not only for ensuring best possible care, but also from a financial perspective: the combination of recommendations on prevention and those for diagnosis and treatment (or general guidelines on factors influencing population health) could contribute to prompt interventions and an overall improvement in health.

The divergent practices regarding the development, dissemination and implementation of clinical guidelines largely reflect the different stages of quality assurance development across health systems. Knowledge exchange in this field already takes place, both informally (with practitioners "borrowing" published guidelines from other countries) and formally (in the form of collaborating networks, such as G-I-N). There is considerable experience in the realm of best practice with collaborating platforms endorsed at a European level: the European Network for Health Technology Assessment (EUnetHTA) programme (EUnetHTA, 2012) has been successful in promoting the optimization of HTA methodology and transfer of knowledge. A similar initiative for clinical guideline development would definitely benefit countries in which related practices are still in their infancy.

The challenges identified by the research presented in this book clearly outline that there is a need to:

- produce a consolidated set of terms and conceptual frameworks for clinical guidelines, which will ensure clear and effective collaboration;

- facilitate knowledge exchange on established methodologies for the development and implementation of clinical guidelines;

- understand how clinical guidelines might need to be contextualized to different countries, to ensure appropriateness of practice;

- invest in developing or enhancing guideline evaluation mechanisms and methodological approaches to enquire into the utilization and effectiveness of clinical guidelines in practice;

- develop strategies for increased involvement of professionals and consumers in the production process (to increase representativeness, transparency and effectiveness of recommendations);

- further promote transparency by providing tools for disclosure of conflicts of interest and how to proceed in the event of such conflicts;

- initiate efforts to incorporate prevention and population health recommendations in guideline production (both in terms of priority setting and with regard to methodology); and

- encompass more actors and thus increase collaboration and awareness (actors identified in the mapping exercise could function as an initial network).

The mapping exercise in Part 2 of this book highlights the lack of properly evaluated information on actual practices in several European countries. Seen in conjunction with this insight, the literature review in Part 4 is especially revealing, illustrating the dearth of rigorous studies that assess the quality and effectiveness of clinical guidelines in Europe. Moreover, there is inconsistency in existing results on the effect of clinical guidelines on process and outcomes of care. Based on these findings, the development of more rigorous studies to evaluate patients' health outcomes associated with the use of clinical guidelines is clearly called for. Furthermore, a comprehensive assessment of the cost–effectiveness of developing, disseminating and implementing clinical guidelines is of particular importance, in order to ensure their appropriate use.

With regard to the guidelines themselves, suggested research priorities should include the careful investigation of the perspectives of service users and staff with respect to clinical guideline development and implementation, using both qualitative and quantitative assessments; and – taking into consideration current gaps in guideline topics – the development of further studies evaluating guidelines on prevention, depressive disorder and other mental health conditions.

Part 6

European country profiles on clinical guidelines

(A list of country profile authors is available at the beginning of the book)

Questionnaire template sent out to authors

This short questionnaire aims at exploring the regulatory basis, actors and their responsibilities regarding the development, implementation and evaluation of clinical guidelines in your country, with such guidelines defined as "systematically developed statements to assist important professional and patient decisions about appropriate health care for specific circumstances". Clinical guidelines aim to describe appropriate care based on the best available evidence as well as on systematic and transparent consensus processes.

We focus initially on six main topics regarding clinical guidelines for chronic conditions (e.g. diabetes, coronary heart disease, asthma/COPD, cancer, arthritis).

Please provide short answers (plus further material, e.g. publications, if relevant) as you will be contacted for further details if appropriate/necessary.

Background: Do clinical guidelines on preventing and/or treating chronic diseases exist in your country (possibly under another name)? If not: (a) Do they exist for other types of diseases or interventions? (b) Are there any other tools to assist professionals and patients in making appropriate decisions for the chronically ill?

Regulatory basis: Is there an "official" basis for clinical guideline development and implementation in your country, e.g. a legal basis (possibly indirectly, e.g. as part of NSFs or Disease Management Programmes), a government document or a statement by an ALB or quasi-official agency (possibly the same as for HTA)? If yes, which? If no, are there any proposals to create it?

Development: Is the process of clinical guideline development carried out centrally (e.g. through an ALB) or is it decentralized (or does it differ for different clinical guidelines, e.g. prevention versus treatment)? If centralized, by whom? If decentralized, by whom (e.g. professional organizations or individual groups of physicians)? Are there guidelines for clinical guideline development (e.g. regarding the grading of the evidence, stakeholder involvement, editorial independence), and if yes, by whom? Is the decentralized process coordinated (e.g. by an association of professional organizations or an ALB)?

Quality control: Are clinical guidelines checked for quality (e.g. using the AGREE instrument) before being implemented, and if yes, by whom (i.e. the same or a different body than that developing clinical guidelines)? Is it a requirement, and if yes, by whom?

Implementation: Is the use of (certain) guidelines mandatory (possibly called differently, e.g. "directives")? If yes, who regulates that? If not mandatory, are there (financial) incentives to implement and use clinical guidelines (e.g. through contracts between purchasers and providers)? Is clinical guideline use promoted through IT applications or other tools?

Evaluation: Is the development, quality control, implementation and use of clinical guidelines (regularly) evaluated, and if yes, by whom and using which criteria? Is it a requirement, and if yes, by whom?

Austria

Background

Clinical guidelines do exist in Austria for all kinds of diseases, and in particular for chronic conditions. Most of these guidelines are being developed within the different national and international societies of medical specialists. However, established medical guidelines for certain diseases or disease groups are almost non-existent at the national level in Austria.

The main regulatory basis in Austrian legislation for the use of clinical guidelines is found in the Physicians' Act, which obliges physicians to pursue continuing medical education, and in the Federal Law on the Quality of Health Care Services (Austrian Federal Health Commission, 2010). This law distinguishes the federal quality (*Bundesqualitätsrichtlinien*), which are legally binding, and the federal quality (*Bundesqualitätsleitlinien*), which are recommendations (not legally binding). Both are issued by the Federal Minister of Health.

Guidelines are federally regulated but other non-official projects also exist for developing them, such as the "Arznei & Vernunft" initiative (Arznei & Vernunft, 2012), which launched a joint project between the Austrian Social Insurance Fund and the pharmaceutical industry to evaluate the cost–effectiveness of drugs, as well as their usefulness and limits for a number of conditions. Arznei & Vernunft publish therapeutic recommendations and patient information brochures on their web site.

Recommendations for general practitioners or internal specialists are also available on the "Verlagshaus der Ärzte" publishing house web site (Verlagshaus der Ärzte, 2012), providing an overview of state-of-the-art diagnoses, therapies and strategies for a large number of conditions.

Regulatory basis

The Federal Institute for Quality Assurance in Health Care (BIQG) was established within the Austrian Health Institute (GmbH) in 2007 to support the Ministry of Health in encouraging high-quality integrated health care through the development of guidelines and standards for process and structural quality. These guidelines do not replace clinical guidelines; instead, they integrate them into broader guidelines which also include recommendations on organizational problems (GÖG, 2012).[8]

The GmbH has recently published a "meta-guideline" method for the development and evaluation of federal quality guidelines (Baumer, Holzer & Wabro, 2010). This methodological guidance has been based on previous international recommendations, such as the AGREE tools, the DELBI tools, the G-I-N and the SIGN. The "meta-guideline" determines the national methodology for developing and implementing federal quality guidelines. This methodology prescribes, for example, that federal quality guidelines do not only need to refer to clinical procedures but should also take into consideration inter-professional work and transition processes between the structures involved (integrated care). Three federal quality guidelines are currently being developed (on dementia, Parkinson's disease, and COPD) and a public consultation is being carried out relating to a guideline for early prevention of breast cancer. However, the Austrian Chamber of Medical Doctors is opposed to the overall idea of federal quality guidelines that are too prescriptive, as they see it as restricting their decision-making regarding the treatment of individual patients.

Development

According to the meta-guideline approach, as part of the development of

8 See also the *Gesundheitsreformgesetz* (Health Care Reform Act) (German Federal Law Gazette, 2004).

the federal quality guidelines, all of the following issues must be considered: principles of nationwide standardization, health service integration, professional relevance, patient-centredness, health promotion, transparency, evidence based on the topic, and experience concerning effectiveness and efficiency. The topic for federal quality guidelines can be suggested by any organization, and priorities are evaluated by a subcommission within the GmbH (the UAG quality sub-working group), in accordance with the Federal Minister of Health. All relevant stakeholders are involved in the development of federal quality guidelines, including patient representatives.

The draft of the guideline must be validated by a pool of experts. Subsequently, the financial impact and feasibility need to be assessed, followed by an external review carried out by means of a consensus process, which involves certain members of the public. The final version is published on the web site.

This procedure also applies when monitoring the quality of existing standards.

Quality control

A validation process exists for the federal quality guidelines. However, in cases in which clinical guidelines are developed by medical associations or expert groups, no quality monitoring mechanism is in place (thus far). The quality and accepted validity of these clinical guidelines can vary quite significantly, depending on the medical society that developed them, and on the use of an international evidence base or related recommendations (for example, from the G-I-N (G-I-N, 2012)).

The only federal quality guideline that has been fully developed and published on the web site of the BMG so far relates to type 2 diabetes mellitus management (BMG, 2009).

In an issue of the *Guidelines* journal published by the Medical Association of Upper Austria, a number of specific guidelines are recommended and a checklist for quality control is provided (Alkin, 2001). In this list, for example, questions on responsibility and authorship of the guideline are raised, as well as questions relating to transparency of the development process, objectives of the guideline, indications of usefulness, side-effects, costs and results, dissemination and implementation. Also, as mentioned earlier, the evidence-based medicine Guidelines web site (Verlagshaus der Ärzte, 2012) and Arznei & Vernunft (2012) provide information on reliable guidelines for diagnoses and treatment pathways.

Implementation

So far only one federal quality guideline has been fully developed and implemented at the national level.

According to the meta-guideline approach, in practice guidelines do not represent binding regulations but should serve as a basis for decision-making as sound and effective tools in patient care. It is acknowledged that deviations (for good reasons) are inevitable in certain cases, and local conditions or the legal framework under which a guideline is implemented should always be taken into account.

Evaluation

With the meta-guideline approach, the effectiveness of federal quality guidelines has to be ensured by the respective organization in charge of launching the development of such guidelines. Not only the guideline's impact on care quality, but also its acceptance and degree of implementation need to be evaluated. The reasons for not implementing a guideline must be documented and analysed, and measures for improvement must be considered when reviewing the guideline. In addition, the meta-guideline approach requires the guideline to include a planned date for evaluation, with specific indicators. As far as possible, such evaluations should be representative and are to be carried out nationally. Funding for evaluation must be provided by the initiators of the guideline.

Belgium

Background

Clinical guidelines on preventing and treating chronic conditions exist in Belgium.

Clinical guidelines used in Belgium can be differentiated as (i) informal consensus-based guidelines (which are developed by a group of experts based on their opinion and practical experience), (ii) formal consensus-based guidelines (developed using systematic methods) and (iii) evidence-based practice guidelines. The latter are developed by a team of clinical and methodological experts, taking into account evidence based on the relevant literature, practical experience, values, preferences and circumstances.

The majority of the clinical guidelines operate at local, regional or national levels. Different entities are involved in clinical guidelines development and implementation. Some clinical guidelines are local revisions of international guidelines, while in other cases international recommendations are distributed without revision (as is the case with arthritis guidelines in Belgium).

Decentralized associations have developed clinical guidelines for some chronic conditions. The Belgian Diabetes Association – a non-official association involving patients, practitioners and academic staff – developed clinical guidelines for type 2 diabetes mellitus based upon European recommendations. The Belgian Society of Cardiology revised international and European recommendations to develop Belgian guidelines on coronary heart disease and the Belgian Society of Pneumology developed clinical guidelines on COPD based on those of the Dutch Society of Pneumology. The College of Oncology – linked with the KCE and aiming to expand the use of evidence-based medicine – developed and disseminated clinical guidelines on the management of several types of cancer. Clinical guidelines are also available for several other chronic conditions.

Regulatory basis

Several structures have been developed with the scope of disseminating the use of clinical guidelines, such as the colleges of physicians, the KCE, the CEBAM, the EBMPracticeNet and the Federal Council for the Quality of Nursing. However, there is no central coordination of guideline development in Belgium; their development can be at the initiative of both governmental and other organizations.

The development, dissemination and evaluation of clinical guidelines related to hospital nursing care are more systematically organized and centralized. The Federal Council for the Quality of Nursing, together with the Federal Public Service (Public Health) and nursing faculties at Belgian universities select, disseminate and implement clinical guidelines on the nursing care of patients with chronic diseases. Currently, 62 clinical guidelines are available in three languages (English, French and Dutch). These guidelines are selected by performing a literature review and quality evaluation of the findings (UGENT & UCL, 2012; FPS, 2012).

Development

Several entities – centralized or not – are involved in the development and dissemination of clinical guidelines, such as universities, professional associations, hospitals, scientific associations, colleges of medicine, and governmental entities.

Clinical guidelines can be either funded by the government, or by the different organizations involved. When clinical guidelines are funded by national and regional authorities, the topics are sometimes chosen by these authorities, while respecting the professional autonomy of the guideline developers.

Since 2009 a voluntary platform of national evidence-based medicine organizations has been working to stimulate cooperation and coordination between the different entities, in order to strengthen the the implementation of clinical guidelines. This platform is due to be transformed into a non-profit-making organization with legal basis (EBMPracticeNet). In this way the National Council for Quality Promotion – which forms part of the National Institute for Health and Disability Insurance (NIHDI) – could play an important role in the methodology of the EBMPracticeNet by determining priorities in developing or updating national guidelines and in the national adaptation of international guidelines.

Within the centralized structured organizations, there is the KCE (KCE, 2011), which has been created in order to promote evidence-based medicine through the evaluation of practices, HTA and guidelines diffusion. In addition, the Belgian Antibiotic Policy Coordination Committee (BAPCOC) is in charge of publishing several clinical guidelines.

Belgium is a member of the G-I-N though the CEBAM and Domus Medica (the Flemish College of General Practitioners). The KCE collaborates with the SIGN to produce literature reviews for specific key questions.

Since the early 2000s the development of clinical guidelines has become more rigorous. Part of the purpose of the EBMPracticeNet is the integration of information from Belgian evidence-based medicine organizations with the information available in the international evidence-based medicine guidelines database, including their adaption where necessary to the local context and their dissemination to Belgian health care professionals.

In 2011 a Flemish working group "Recommendations" was also set up to bring guideline developers together at regional level.

Although clinical guidelines have become more evidence-based medicine focused in Belgium, the way in which they are developed is not standardized across the country. The composition of the GDGs differs across the different clinical guidelines and the different organizations. Usually the main participants are clinicians, content experts, and systematic review experts. In governmental settings, policy-makers and health economists can also be included. For some very specific guidelines, patient representatives are also being included. Moreover, the methodology for clinical guidelines development also varies across the organizations, along with the approach for retrieving and assessing evidence-based medicine practices. In general the critical appraisal of evidence is carried out by researchers or health care professionals with relevant skills acquired through specific training or education. The CEBAM provides training in evidence-based medicine.

Quality control

Validation of clinical guidelines is not mandatory and there is no standard procedure for this. The organization that developed the clinical guidelines is responsible for their validation, at the request of the guideline authors. If requested, the CEBAM validates guidelines with the AGREE instrument in combination with a limited analysis of the content. The validation procedure results in a decision by the targeted caregivers to recommend or not to recommend the use of the guideline. Sometimes this step is a prerequisite for funding from the government, for example for clinical guidelines proposed by the KCE.

All guidelines in the field of nursing must be evaluated on the basis of four criteria: AGREE, Cluzeau, Grilli, & Shaneyfelt. Evaluations are provided by universities, and the results are published, receiving a global score for their quality.

The dissemination of the clinical guidelines is not standardized. The organization that develops them is also responsible for their publication. Belgian scientific associations and colleges of physicians disseminate their clinical guidelines through their professional papers or in the medical local press. In addition, a web site has been launched, which provides access to a broad range of national and international evidence-based medicine approaches (CEBAM Digital Library for Health (2012)) and the EBMPracticeNet also represents a new channel for disseminating guidelines.

Clinical guidelines that have been adapted from other countries or areas are usually tested for applicability in the Belgian context according to the ADAPTE instrument, which is used by various organizations.

Implementation

The use of guidelines is not mandatory for physicians – there is only a legal basis for the implementation of clinical guidelines in hospitals for nursing. However, the access to some drugs, therapeutic measures or diagnostic interventions can be subject to compliance to guidelines. Moreover, quality evaluations of hospital nursing care are based upon indicators contained within the guidelines.

The implementation of clinical guidelines is not standardized. Multifaceted interventions are advocated and a number of different types of tools are being used, including care protocols and clinical pathways. A new tool to be introduced is the EBMeDS system, which brings evidence into practice by means of context-sensitive guidance at the point of care through the electronic patient record.

Evaluation

Currently no formal data exist concerning the extent to which clinical guidelines are used in Belgium. Generally their use is not monitored, apart from selected specific topics (such as antibiotics).

A new system is being developed for evaluating hospital nursing clinical guidelines; initial results are expected in 2014. Some colleges of physicians also define criteria for clinical guideline evaluations and assess them; however, this is not carried out systematically.

Bulgaria

Background

The process of registration, monitoring and treatment of chronic diseases in Bulgaria is subject to a special regulation issued by the Ministry of Health (Bulgarian Ministry of Health, 2008). It describes all the chronic diseases that are subject to "dispensarization", which is provided either by a general practitioner or a related specialist or in hospitals.[9] The latter provide acute care or rehabilitation to chronic patients. The overall system for managing chronic conditions in Bulgaria is not integrated, since different health care providers work independently from each other and do not have common responsibilities in managing care. Their interaction for the same patient is mostly based on the exchange of medical documentation.

Similarly to this disintegrated system, clinical guidelines on chronic diseases refer to separate episodes of illness and do not embrace the overall process of managing the condition. Bearing in mind the definition of clinical guidelines used in this report, few of the recommendations existing in Bulgaria completely satisfy the clinical guidelines requirements. Many of the existing recommendations (see the different types in the subsections that follow) aim to predetermine physicians' behaviour rather than to support the appropriate decision-making process.

---

9 For chronic conditions, these are the former "dispensaries", now called mental health centres, comprehensive cancer centres and centres for dermato-venereal conditions.

Regulatory basis

There is a legal basis for the development and implementation of centrally developed regulations. For example, the development and implementation of the national medical standards (NMS) is regulated by the 2004 Law on Health. There is no legal basis for guidelines produced by associations and societies.

Development

One form of clinical guidelines employed in Bulgaria is the clinical pathways[10] used by the National Health Insurance Fund[11] as an instrument for hospital care financing. Some clinical pathways describe the treatment of acute episodes of chronic conditions; others refer to rehabilitation for chronic patients. Another form of clinical guidelines takes the form of National Health Insurance Fund requirements for the volume and type of activities, as well as diagnostic tests that physicians must provide to chronic patients included in their list for "dispensary monitoring". These requirements include a description of the illness, the required length and frequency of monitoring, specialized medical activities, and the required consultation and diagnostic tests by type and volume. Based on the 2004 Law on Health, 56 NMSs for different specialties have been developed since 2011 (Bulgarian Ministry of Health, 2009). These include aspects such as professional activities, quality criteria and conditions to protect medical professionals during their practice (Bulgarian Ministry of Health, 2008). Some parts of the NMS are similar to clinical guidelines in purpose and various elements of their composition. For example, the NMS "Endocrinology and metabolic diseases" includes an algorithm which general practitioners and endocrinologists are obliged to follow while managing diabetes.

For specific conditions the Ministry of Health issues methodological guidance, for example on the referral, diagnosis, monitoring, and treatment of patients with latent tuberculosis and on antiretroviral treatment and monitoring of adults with HIV infection. These are typical clinical guidelines as defined in this report, but their volume is limited and does not encompass all chronic conditions. Scientific medical associations and academic societies develop clinical guidelines, algorithms and protocols based on Bulgarian publications in recognized international journals. They are not mandatory and their implementation depends on the provider.

---

10 According to Bulgarian legislation, "clinical pathway" is a system of requirements and guidelines for diagnostic and therapeutic procedures for patients with certain diseases requiring hospitalization.

11 The National Health Insurance Fund is the only social health insurance fund in Bulgaria. Most hospital financing comes from the National Health Insurance Fund.

All legally regulated guidelines are developed centrally. The National Health Insurance Fund is responsible for the development of clinical pathways, while Ministry of Health experts develop NMS and methodological guidelines.

Quality control

All guidelines are developed by means of consensus processes, supported by current literature. Clinical pathways, as well as the NMS, have been periodically updated during the implementation process. Updates are often initiated by medical professionals, but the Ministry of Health and the National Health Insurance Fund are responsible for guideline quality.

Implementation

The implementation of the NMS is mandatory for all health care providers. Implementation is controlled by the regional structures of the Ministry of Health – the Regional Health Inspections. Clinical pathways are mandatory for all hospitals contracted by the National Health Insurance Fund: in order to receive payment, requirements and guidelines included in the pathway must be strictly followed. The same applies to general practitioners and outpatient specialist providers funded by the National Health Insurance Fund.

Evaluation

In terms of population health improvement or the effectiveness of recommendations, there is no evidence that such evaluation is performed. One of the reasons for this is that these instruments are used as a method of financing, rather than as a method for quality improvement. The National Health Insurance Fund controls provider compliance with contractual agreements. Professional medical societies carry out scientific research on the effectiveness of using clinical guidelines and algorithms.

Cyprus

Background

Clinical guidelines on preventing and treating chronic disease do exist in Cyprus. However, they are poorly implemented and their implementation is inadequately assessed. At the moment there are no other tools available to assist professionals in making appropriate decisions for chronically ill patients.

However, the new NHIS includes a specific proposal to improve the whole process of developing, implementing and evaluating clinical guidelines. These new tools have not yet been put into practice.

Regulatory basis

There is no official basis for clinical guidelines development and implementation in Cyprus; that is, the legal basis is lacking.

Development

The responsible body for developing and implementing clinical guidelines in Cyprus is the Ministry of Health. A parallel role has now been taken up by the National Health Insurance Organization, which is responsible for implementing the new NHIS.

Committees have been developed to evaluate the relevant clinical guidelines for the different medical specialties. A significant number of clinical guidelines are in the process of being finalized. Unfortunately, the development of clinical guidelines is not carried out through evidence-based methodology.

Quality control

Currently, clinical guidelines are not checked for quality before being implemented. Changes in the process and quality control of the development/implementation, adaptation and evaluation of clinical guidelines are being discussed; however, these changes have not yet been effected.

Implementation

The use of clinical guidelines is not mandatory and there are no financial incentives for their implementation and use. However, the new NHIS includes the use of financial incentives to maximize clinical guidelines implementation and adherence, as well as new tools to promote the dissemination of clinical guidelines through IT applications. Specifically, the development of an electronic disease management system is planned, to support physicians through the decision-making process for specific chronic diseases.

Evaluation

Currently, no evaluation processes are in place to evaluate the implementation and use of clinical guidelines. Tools for evaluating guidelines implementation have been proposed within the new NHIS.

Czech Republic

Background

Clinical practice guidelines do exist and have been periodically updated in the Czech Republic for the following chronic conditions: diabetes, coronary heart disease, asthma, COPD, and cancer. In addition, to varying degrees of sophistication over 250 clinical practice guidelines have been published since 2006 (and are periodically revised and updated) (Forýtková & Bourek, 2006, 2008). Several web portals exist to assist professionals and patients in making appropriate decisions where care for the chronically ill is required, but the majority of these portals are not systematically maintained and developed.

Regulatory basis

Since 2009 the National Reference Centre (NRC) has been in charge of developing methodologies and implementing development of the National Set of Healthcare Standards (NSHS) and of the National Healthcare Services Indicator Set (NHSIS). A joint development of both these national sets of standards is being implemented to establish uniform, standardized tools for improving the quality of care in the Czech health care system.

Development

The process of clinical guideline development is centralized; the NRC (NRC, 2012) is in charge of the development of national sets of clinical guidelines and quality indicators since 2006. It belongs to (and is financed by) the Ministry of Health. There is also a decentralized branch, represented by DASHOFER publishing house, funded by external resources and coordinated by the Center for Healthcare Quality at the Masaryk University Faculty of Medicine.

The two entities collaborate in developing clinical guidelines. However, there is no formally defined and nationally accepted guidance for the development of clinical guidelines.

Quality control

The AGREE instrument is widely used for the purpose of quality control. For the main standards, quality control is undertaken by professional medical associations (Czech Medical Association of J.E. Purkyně).

Implementation

The implementation and use of clinical guidelines is not mandatory. Assessment of adherence to clinical guidelines is self-organized. Clinical guidelines are strongly promoted through IT applications.

Evaluation

The evaluation of clinical guidelines is currently being developed.

Denmark

Background

In Denmark, clinical guidelines are provided for a range of conditions and there has been an increased emphasis on preventing and treating chronic diseases. Data are not available about other tools assisting professionals and patients in making appropriate decisions for chronic diseases, although such tools are in place in the Danish health care system.

Regulatory basis

The Health Act stated that the National Board of Health is authorized to develop clinical guidelines. Traditionally, however, medical societies also participate, along with professional organizations and, due to the general operational responsibility, local authorities.

Development

Clinical guidelines are developed at both central and decentralized levels. The National Board of Health, as the supreme professional health care authority, and the Institute for Rational Pharmacotherapy provide guidance at a central level. Regional and municipal authorities, professional organizations, nursing associations and medical societies also develop clinical guidelines. Notably, the Danish College of General Practitioners (DSAM) is involved in two ways; by producing its own guidelines and by participating in the development of central ones. There is no general guide for preparing, developing and implementing clinical guidelines. Moreover, there is no single institution to coordinate the clinical guideline development process.

Quality control

Although clinical guidelines normally need to meet international standards, there's no formalized requirement for a quality assessment ahead of implementation. The AGREE instrument is often used to assess clinical guideline quality when guidelines are used for HTA production.[12]

Implementation

No law is currently in place mandating practitioners to follow clinical guidelines, but due diligence on behalf of health care professionals regulates their practices (based on the assumption that practitioners keep themselves informed and follow best practice – *ergo* clinical guidelines). Furthermore, professionals are often supported by different IT applications as well as through Disease Management Programmes. A recent study by Carlsen & Kjellberg (2010) shows that general practitioners in Denmark have encountered difficulties accessing guidelines, attributing low utilization – to some extent – to a lack of a unified platform for evidence seeking (that is, no guideline database is available).

Evaluation

The development, quality control, implementation and use of clinical guidelines are evaluated within accreditation programmes for publicly funded hospitals.

Estonia

Background

Several clinical guidelines are available in Estonia, including those for the management of chronic conditions. Professional medical associations have been increasingly developing clinical guidelines either *ex novo* or by translating foreign guidelines. Sometimes there may be several guidelines for one condition. Some are formally acknowledged by the single public payer – the Estonian Health Insurance Fund (EHIF) (EHIF, 2012) – but this number remains relatively low. Other tools (for example, white papers for home, school or family nurses) are also available to assist professionals.

Regulatory basis

The EHIF highlights the need for good clinical quality in the contracts made with providers. In 2003, professional medical societies and the EHIF formed an agreement, according to which a number of public institutions within the health system (the EHIF, the Ministry of Social Affairs, the National Institute for Health Development, the Estonian e-Health Foundation, providers of

---

12 DACEHTA is the main authority for HTA production in Denmark.

health care services, various medical associations, and so on) have certain mandates to facilitate or/and develop clinical guidelines.

Development

The vast majority of current clinical guidelines have been developed by professional associations and many of those were commissioned by the EHIF, which has been coordinating development methodologies since 2003. The handbook on clinical guideline methodology was updated in accordance with WHO standards in 2011 (Bero et al., 2012). In addition, both the Ministry of Social Affairs and the National Institute for Health Development have recently commissioned a limited amount of guidelines. Best practice is further endorsed by individual health care providers using their own treatment practices, patient guidelines or pathways.

Quality control

The quality of developed guidelines is safeguarded by the aforementioned methodological handbook and a guideline adoption procedure stipulated in the memorandum agreed by the EHIF and the relevant professional societies. Both the handbook and the adoption procedures were reviewed and updated in 2011 (Bero et al., 2012).

Implementation

There is no formal legal basis for clinical guidelines in Estonia; only a vague obligation to implement "guidelines for good clinical practice" as part of the responsibility of each individual health care provider (based on a regulation of the Ministry of Social Affairs). The importance of following clinical guidelines is highlighted in the contracts between providers (both primary care and hospitals) and the EHIF, and monitored during clinical audits and by the "trustee doctors" system that functions within the insurance system. However, the limited number and low specificity of existing guidelines results in them being used more as evidence sources than as conclusive treatment recommendations.

A bonus payment system for quality improvement has been implemented in family medicine in Estonia since 2005. It includes indicators on chronic conditions (such as hypertension and diabetes) and prevention/promotion (such as child care and vaccinations). These indicators are developed based on examples of good clinical practices and their respective guidelines. Currently, no IT applications support guideline consideration in everyday practice.

Evaluation

Currently no evaluation system exists in Estonia. A discussion among experts has been initiated.

Finland

Background

Clinical guidelines are developed by the Duodecim, a scientific association which works to develop the professional skills of physicians and support their clinical practice with further education, publications and research grants. The *Käypä hoito* (Current Care) Unit drafts nationwide care guidelines to improve the quality of care and reduce variations in care practices. The guidelines are designed to support physicians in their clinical practice and for the benefit of the patient, serving as the basis for drafting regional treatment pathways (Duodecim, 2011b).

National clinical guidelines exist, focusing on over 100 clinical conditions, many of them dealing with chronic conditions (such as diabetes, asthma, rheumatic disease, and a range of cancers). Most clinical guidelines focus on prevention, and all on treatment. The clinical guidelines support doctors' practical work and form a basis for compiling regional care programmes. Furthermore, these guidelines are applicable to medical practice in Finland. As such, they may also include well-founded comments on significant health care issues for which no scientific evidence is available. The clinical guidelines can be used to improve the quality of care and reduce inconsistencies between treatment practices. The clinical guidelines are also integrated with the EBMeDS system, allowing clinical guidelines to be accessed from within the electronic patient record.

The Current Care Unit and the Duodecim are founding members of the G-I-N (G-I-N, 2012).

Regulatory basis

Clinical guidelines in Finland are produced by the Duodecim, and thus they have no direct legal basis. However, they are mainly funded by the Finnish Government, via the THL, which is a governmental organization. The government also strongly supports their implementation.

Development

The Current Care Editorial Office is led by a Board comprising 15 members, representing a range of interest groups and Duodecim's management team. The editorial staff includes part-time editing doctors or "Current Care editors", as well as information specialists, technical editors participating in content production, and editing staff compiling patient versions of information and educational material. The process of clinical guideline development is conducted centrally by the Duodecim. The in-house manual for guideline development, produced and maintained by the Duodecim, is based mainly on the "GRADE" and "AGREE" methods and standards.

Quality control

The Current Care Board selects the topics to be covered by clinical guidelines, mainly based on suggestions made by specialist societies. These specialist societies operate as the host associations for the guideline in question, in partnership with the Duodecim. The "PRIO-tool" – or a set of criteria for assessing the guideline topic proposal – is used for prioritizing new guideline topics (Duodecim, 2011a). A systematic review of the literature on the identified topic is first conducted by an experienced professional information specialist. Current Care working groups (including approximately 700 top volunteer health care professionals from a range of fields across Finland) then produce the evidence-based clinical guideline in cooperation with Current Care editors, who operate as method experts. Prior to its completion, the guideline is circulated to specific interest groups for their critical consideration of the content and structure of the clinical guideline, according to the AGREE criteria. Any resulting comments are then discussed and the guideline is revised if required. The completed clinical guidelines and subsequent updates are communicated as appropriate.

Implementation

The use of clinical guidelines is not mandatory and there are no financial incentives encouraging their use. They are not intended to replace the assessment of a doctor or other health care professional in terms of establishing the best possible diagnostics and treatment of an individual patient when making care decisions. Guidelines are widely used in primary care because of their accessibility. The use of clinical guidelines is strongly promoted through IT applications (Duodecim, 2012). Moreover, to support the implementation of clinical guidelines, summaries, patient versions, PowerPoint slide series and online courses are developed (selectively).

Evaluation

Until recently, clinical guidelines were not regularly evaluated. However, since 2011, the THL (THL, 2012) is responsible for supervising the development, quality and use of clinical guidelines.

France

Background

Specific clinical practice guidelines are in place for most diseases and especially for chronic diseases in France. All the developed guidelines are available on the web site of the HAS (HAS, 2012) or the web site of the AFSSAPS (AFSSAPS, 2012).

Regulatory basis

The HAS is an independent scientific public authority aiming, among other things, to promote good practice within the French health care system. The institution of clinical guidelines is established by law as part of the outputs of the HAS (Clerc et al., 2011) Loi du 13 août 2004 relative à l'assurance maladie, Titre II, Chapitre Ier bis, article L. 161-37; it develops, disseminates and evaluates the implementation of clinical guidelines.

Development

Three tiers of clinical guidelines development exist: centrally, undertaken by the HAS; regionally, by regional authorities for some conditions; and by individual providers in certain cases. The HAS publishes its methodology for developing clinical guidelines on its web site. According to the document, the GDG consists of 15–20 specialists from different disciplines related to the topic, as well as representatives of the patients and/or health system users. The formulation of recommendations is based on a literature review on behalf of the development team. Once synthesized, the recommendations are reviewed by a group of 30–50 people (with a composition similar to that of the GDG) and feedback is provided, upon which the recommendations are modified accordingly. The HAS aims at maximum transparency and objectivity by making both the development and the review group as independent as possible, both editorially and in terms of conflict of interest.

Quality control

The Guidelines Commission (Commission Recommendations) as well as the

College de la HAS validates the recommendations before the guidelines are published on the agency's web site. An evidence grading system – based on study design – is used in the guidelines to underpin the evidence base of each recommendation.

Implementation

HAS guidance is disseminated by use of the agency's web site and potentially also by auxiliary scientific publications and presentations at relevant congresses. Guidelines are not mandatory (an initial phase of financial penalties for non-compliance was soon abandoned). A recent study shows that awareness among practitioners is not particularly high and more active implementation would be necessary to achieve a higher rate of guideline application (Clerc et al., 2011). General practitioners do have to follow Professional Practice Assessments, during which they are made aware of guidelines and are required to compare their practice to them.

Evaluation

The HAS clinical guideline methodology foresees that the agency keeps abreast of developments, so as to be able to initiate guideline updates if research emerges that suggests a significant deviation from existing recommendations. Given that guidelines are not mandatory, no official mechanism for evaluation is in place as yet.

Germany

Background

In Germany, clinical guidelines are produced on a multitude of conditions, including the prevention and treatment of chronic diseases. Chronic diseases in particular have been the target of Disease Management Programmes (ÄZQ, 2010), which have been implemented nationwide by the statutory health insurance funds in recent years (for breast cancer and TD2M since 2002; for coronary heart disease and chronic heart failure due to coronary heart disease since 2003 and 2009, respectively; and for asthma and COPD since 2005). Also, the AQUA Institute (2012b) endorses the use of related quality indicators on behalf of providers. In June 2011 the database of the AWMF (AWMF, 2012a) contained 679 clinical guidelines. Guidelines are also collected by the German e-Health library, *Arztbibliothek* (ÄZQ, 2011a).

Regulatory basis

The AWMF (the umbrella organization of 158 medical societies) has been coordinating the development of clinical guidelines on behalf of the medical associations in Germany since 1995 (AWMF, 2012a). A separate kind of guidelines – the NVL programme forms the basis for Disease Management Programmes in Germany and are coordinated by the AWMF and the BÄK, in cooperation with the KBV via their joint institute (the ÄZQ). These institutions agreed on national standards for guideline production and implementation, based on the Council of Europe Recommendation Rec(2001)13 (Council of Europe, 2001). The utilization of evidence-based guidelines is also firmly rooted in the Social Security Statute V, which delineates the code of conduct for statutory health insurance.

Development

The process of guideline development in Germany is carried out both centrally and at a decentralized level. The centralized guidelines of the NVL programme are those of the BÄK, the KBV (at the ÄZQ) and the AWMF (ÄZQ, 2009), the guidelines of the BÄK Scientific Advisory Board (BÄK Scientific Advisory Board, 2010), as well as the Therapy Guidelines of the BÄK Drug Commission (AkdÄ, 2012). Decentralized guidelines developed by the scientific medical societies are coordinated by the AWMF (AWMF, 2012a). The NVL programme has its own guidance manual, while the AWMF and the ÄZQ provide a detailed handbook for decentralized guideline production (AWMF & ÄZQ, 2000).

Quality control

Guidelines coordinated by the ÄZQ or AWMF are checked for quality before being implemented within the framework of the *Arztbibliothek*. The appraisal is carried out by means of the DELBI checklist (ÄZQ, 2011b). DELBI is based on the AGREE I instrument and adapted to the specific setting of the German health care system. The appraisal is performed by methodologists who were not part of the guideline production process. The AWMF categorizes guidelines based on their methodological background using the so-called S-classification (with S1 being the lowest, drawing on expert opinion, and S3 being the highest, designating a guideline which is based on evidence and consensus process; see also Muche-Borowski & Kopp (2011)).

Implementation

There is no definitive legal requirement for the utilization of guidelines in

Germany. However, whether or not treatment was carried out according to official guidelines can be used as an argument during malpractice cases (Berndt & Fischer, 2000). Financial incentives to implement guidelines are used increasingly, especially as part of Disease Management Programme contracts between social insurance institutions and health care providers. Other tools for guideline implementation that exist include quality indicator programmes, such as the Program for Cross-Sectoral Quality Assurance of the Federal Joint Committee at the AQUA Institute (AQUA Institute, 2012a). Hospitals are increasingly combining IT applications with clinical pathways based on clinical guidelines. This development is still in its infancy in the outpatient care setting.

Evaluation

No overarching national agenda exists on evaluating the implementation and use of clinical guidelines. The National Academy of Family Physicians regularly evaluates all guidelines within its scope. The development and quality of guidelines coordinated by the AWMF and ÄZQ are regularly evaluated by these organizations, using the aforementioned instruments. The implementation and utilization of clinical guidelines are evaluated within the setting of disease management contracts and of guideline-based quality indicator programmes. The IQWiG has been mandated by the G-BA to systematically research and evaluate current guidelines (both German and international) in order to pinpoint the necessity for updating the regulations underpinning Disease Management Programmes in Germany (see the Diabetes case study relating to Germany in Part 3 of this report).

Greece

Background

Strictly speaking, clinical guidelines are still at an early stage of development in Greece. Recommendations by specialist medical societies exist for diabetes, coronary heart disease, asthma/COPD (primary care) and rheumatoid arthritis (in Greek). Clinical guidelines developed in other countries (in English) are available on local medical societies' web sites. Professionals depend to a great extent on their individual efforts to gather the appropriate evidence in order to make informed decisions. Several sets of terminology for these processes are used by professionals, including "clinical practices" or "clinical protocols".

Regulatory basis

There is no official basis for the development or implementation of clinical guidelines.

Development

No process exists for clinical guidelines development in Greece. Discussion is under way to decide who is going to be responsible for developing clinical guidelines.

Quality control

There is no uniform process for quality control, as guideline initiatives themselves are sporadic. In terms of quality control of the clinical guidelines for diabetes, the ADA and the SIGN evaluation systems have been used. For coronary heart disease, the ESCARDIO CPG evaluation system is used and for the asthma/COPD clinical guidelines (in primary care), the IPCRG evaluation system is used. The AGREE instrument is available (translated into Greek) but it is not reported as a tool in the final edition of the clinical guidelines.

Implementation

The use of clinical guidelines is not mandatory and there are no financial incentives related to their use in Greece. Individual clinical guideline initiatives are promoted via web sites, specific congresses and scientific societies. Generally speaking, no IT applications are used to promote the implementation of clinical guidelines. The use of specific clinical guidelines by Greek hospitals depends to a large extent on the medical director of each clinic.

Evaluation

No formal evaluation is undertaken of the implementation of or adherence to clinical guidelines. Research carried out on operating theatres showed that 49% of Greek hospitals have some form of practice guidelines, of which only 51% have applied these to a satisfactory level (Dousis et al., 2008).

Hungary

Background

In Hungary clinical guidelines do exist on preventing and treating chronic conditions as well as on other diseases. Clinical guidelines are produced by each provider (hospital) individually, but on the basis of centralized administration.

Two new organizations are currently the main actors at the central level: the NABHC and the GYEMSZI, both active in this field since 2011. In addition, professional standards assist practitioners in their decision-making processes.

Regulatory basis

No specific law clearly regulates the production and implementation of guidelines. However, the Semmelweis Plan – passed in May 2011 – makes some provisions on quality assurance that may also be useful in this respect (National Institute for Strategic Health Research, 2011).

Development

The Hungarian guideline system has both centralized and decentralized components: based on the condition in question, the NABHC provides treatment recommendations or treatment protocols. Providers (hospitals) are then responsible for formulating actual clinical guidelines for use in their own establishment. Since March 2011, the NABHC has supervised the development and utilization of these guidelines by each specialty and determined the validity period of the guidelines (it has one department for each medical field/specialty, which is responsible, among other things, for guideline supervision).

Protocols include a short introduction to the disease; prevalence/incidence data for Hungary in recent years; as well as information on symptoms, prevention, diagnosis, obligatory and additional examinations, administration documentation, steps and principles of treatment, rehabilitation, and so on.

The NABHC is responsible for professional standards.

Quality control

Quality control of protocols is carried out by the GYEMSZI. The AGREE instrument is also used, for quality assurance. The GYEMSZI is currently developing a methodological guide to enhance and unify protocols and clinical guidelines.

Implementation

Once clinical guidelines have been formulated they are mandatory within the establishment in question.

Evaluation

A partnership is currently in place between the NABHC and the GYEMSZI, with the intention of setting up evaluation processes in the sector.

Ireland

Background

Ireland does not have a comprehensive suite of clinical guidelines but uses international guidance for many of the services that are delivered. However, this is carried out only on an ad hoc basis at present. Examples of specific guidelines and standards include those for symptomatic breast care and health care-associated infections. These guidelines have been mandated through the HIQA (HIQA, 2012), a statutory body charged with regulating and inspecting health care services in Ireland.

The HSE is now rolling out a series of programmes at national level, each with a clinical director and each specifically tasked with improving and standardizing care across health care services. Programmes exist for diabetes, stroke, acute medicine, elective surgery and so on. As part of its functions, each programme will provide a specific set of guidelines, agreed with clinical staff and providing a foundation for normalizing care nationally. These programmes are at an advanced stage of design and an early stage of implementation.

Regulatory basis

The National Clinical Effectiveness Committee (NCEC) has been set up by the Department of Health with the intention of (i) agreeing and mandating a common approach to the development of guidelines in health care nationally; (ii) agreeing guidance and the approach to clinical audit nationally; and (iii) achieving buy-in from all stakeholders on both of the aforementioned items. The Committee is in the process of endorsing a modified AGREE 2 tool for the development of guidelines for health care (with emphasis on common and chronic conditions).

Under the operational wing of the HSE, a number of clinical care programmes exist, each leading the way with fundamental changes and improvements within their own areas, including acute medicine, heart failure, COPD, asthma, acute coronary syndrome, diabetes, health care-associated infections, epilepsy, obstetrics and gynaecology, and acute care surgery. Each of the 30 programmes has a national clinical leader and an administrative manager. Funding is provided for individual projects, including national guidelines. Participation in the projects by individual hospitals is currently voluntary.

The HIQA has the legislative power to investigate failures in care provision and to suspend service delivery. It reports directly to the Minister for Health. Public awareness, confidence and trust in the "HIQA brand" are high, and all HIQA reports are published – leading to a high level of responsiveness within the health service.

Development

As described earlier, the clinical care programmes are advancing in tandem with the work of the NCEC. When combined with the regulatory/investigative role of the HIQA, the multiplicity of levers is having a positive effect on the health care system generally. In addition, a process of rationalization of care delivery centres is under way in Ireland (primarily under the aegis of the National Cancer Control Programme), whereby designated centres are being supported, with care centralized into those centres; this has the additional benefit of ensuring that care follows best practice.

The national care programmes are led by clinical staff who are highly influential amongst their colleagues and nationally esteemed. Each programme is being appropriately funded, even within the constraints of the current economic difficulties and, essentially, the programmes are "the only game in town", so buy-in is accelerated.

Professional competence programmes have become mandatory for medical staff since 2011. All doctors are required to sign up to a college-managed assurance scheme – resulting in heightened awareness of best practice, and increased standardization and clinical guideline adoption.

Quality control

In July 2011 the HIQA published draft guidance on quality criteria for clinical guidelines, to support the development of high-quality clinical guidelines, which includes the AGREE II tool, adapted specifically to the Irish context (HIQA, 2011).

Implementation

Clinical guidelines are not mandatory yet, and licensing for health care organizations is likely to be introduced in the future. All private health care hospitals are required to be accredited with an international accreditation body in order for payments to be forthcoming.

Evaluation

The implementation and use of clinical guidelines are not regularly evaluated.

Italy

Background

Clinical practice guidelines exist for several chronic conditions, such as diabetes, coronary heart disease, COPD, asthma, arthritis, mental health (schizophrenia, autism), thyroid diseases, dementia and epilepsy. Moreover, a number of clinical guidelines exist on acute conditions, emergencies, and elderly care, along with surgical procedures, public health topics and maternal health (ISS-SNLG, 2009).

The updating and development of clinical guidelines and controlled centrally by the SNLG. Among the duties of the SNGL are the updating of existing clinical guidelines and the creation of new ones; the promotion of forums involving different stakeholders (including the patients' associations) to discuss and disseminate clinical guidelines (including versions for laypeople); the training of medical practitioners on using the clinical guidelines; the training of health workers on evidence-based medicine; promoting the implementation of clinical guidelines and collaboration with the regions on evaluating the guidelines.

Regulatory basis

The development of clinical guidelines and their implementation are regulated by the Ministry of Health through the SNLG. This was developed in 2006 with the intention of promoting the elaboration of guidelines on more relevant clinical topics, as well as their evaluation. The SNLG is part of the National Institute of Health (*Istituto Superiore di Sanità* (ISS), a branch of the Ministry of Health) and it collaborates with the Italian Cochrane Centre and with two regional health services (the health system in Italy is run locally by the regions, which have a degree of autonomy).

Development

Clinical guidelines in Italy are developed centrally by the SNLG in collaboration with universities, scientific associations, professional associations and Regional Agencies and Departments of Health. National clinical guidelines are also developed by specialty societies and scientific multi-specialty committees by adapting international clinical guidelines to the local context (for example, clinical guidelines on stroke developed by SPREAD, the Italian guidelines for

COPD, rhinitis and asthma adapted from the international clinical guidelines on rhinitis, asthma and COPD) (Libra, 2002). Local clinical guidelines are also developed by the Regional Agencies. One of the regional offices mainly involved in the development of clinical guidelines is the CeVeAs, located in Modena (CeVeAs, 2012a).

Clinical guidelines are developed on the basis of a practical guide designed by SNLG and available on their web site (ISS-SNLG, 2002). This guide has been designed according to the AGREE standards and defines the methodology in detail, including the process for performing systematic reviews; grading the evidence; monitoring indicators, economical and ethical issues related to the clinical guidelines; and outlining strategies to implement clinical guidelines and evaluate them.

The clinical guidelines are publicly available online on the ISS-SNLG web site (ISS-SNLG, 2009) and the CeVeAs web site (CeVeAs, 2012b).

Quality control

Quality control of clinical guidelines has been a legal requirement since 1992. Clinical guidelines undergo quality control by means of the AGREE instrument, before being implemented. Quality control is assured by the same body/agencies that developed and implemented them (SNLG or CeVeAs), but there is also a dedicated agency responsible for quality control: the AGENAS (AGENAS, 2012b).

In addition, the Italian Society for Quality in Healthcare (SIQuAS-VRQ) (SIQuAS, 2012) is responsible for clinical guidelines quality control. This is the Italian representative of the International Society of Quality in Healthcare (ISQuA) and of the European Society of Quality in Healthcare (ESQH). The SIQuAS-VRQ works in collaboration with the quality offices of hospitals and regional health departments.

Implementation

The use of clinical guidelines is not mandatory in Italy and there are no direct financial incentives for their use. However, some specific directives (known as "Protocols") exist, adherence to which is mandatory; these may be designed by local health institutions (such as hospitals) or by regional health institutions. In the latter case they are mandatory for every medical institute in the region. Protocols are common in the occupational health field (for example, for accidental needle puncture) and for infectious disease control.

National and regional health institutions finance and support targeted implementation projects at hospital and primary care levels in the different regions. The CeVeAs is involved in several of those programmes. The support that these institutions provide includes an analysis of the barriers to implementation and integration of the clinical guidelines into clinical practice, the development of targeted interventions to overcome these barriers, and the resulting evaluation.

Implementation and use of clinical guidelines are also promoted through a special platform called GOAL (ISS-SNLG, 2012), developed by the ISS.

Other organizations are also involved in promoting the implementation and use of clinical guidelines, such as the National Association of Italian General Practitioner Trainees and Young General Practitioners (the Giotto Movement) (Giotto Movement, 2012).

Evaluation

Evaluation of adherence to clinical guidelines is required by law and the AGENAS is in charge of this. It promotes and coordinates special programmes in collaboration with the different regional health care systems (for example, the *Indicators for the evaluation of adherence to the guidelines – manual for companies* (ISS-SNLG, 2007)).

Latvia

Background

Latvia has several clinical guidelines for managing chronic conditions, for example, guidelines for diabetes mellitus types 1 and 2, for COPD in primary care, for the treatment of autoimmune inflammatory arthritis, for the early detection of malignant tumours by general practitioners, for palliative care and for the management of haemophilic patients.

Regulatory basis

There is an official legal basis for both the development and the implementation of clinical guidelines in Latvia. In 2009 the Cabinet of Ministers of the Republic of Latvia published Regulation No. 469 ("Procedures for the development, evaluation, registration and implementation of clinical guidelines"), which was adopted in 2010. The scope of this regulation is the improvement of the quality of guidelines that cover any aspect of health care (such as medical treatment, programmes for medical education, costing and reimbursement, and quality control of health services). The regulation prescribes the procedures for development, evaluation, registration and implementation of guidelines.

Regulation No. 469 prescribes that professional organizations, medical institutions and institutions of higher education which implement academic and professional programmes in medicine have the possibility to draft a clinical guidelines project and submit it to the NHS for approval. The submitted information must contain information about the project's development, identifying information about the author, reviewers, and any discussion that has taken place within the professional organization, medical and scientific institutions, seminars or conferences. The NHS (state institution directly supervised by the Ministry of Health) prepares a list of clinical guidelines, evaluates them and oversees their implementation. Clinical guidelines are publicly accessible on the NHS web site (Latvian NHS, 2012).

The Medical Treatment Law prescribes that medical treatment shall be carried out in conformity with clinical guidelines, taking into account medical principles based upon evidence. The Health Inspectorate, a state administrative institution directly supervised by the Ministry of Health monitors and controls implementation of the laws and regulations that bind health care institutions in the field of health care, including carrying out capacity checks at health care institutions and assessing the quality of professional health care services. The use of drugs and medical treatment is regulated by evaluations of the safety and effectiveness of the drugs, according to an evidence-based medicine approach.

Development

Regulation No. 469 describes and regulates the development of guidelines. These are not detailed methodological guidelines but they meet the minimal requirements regarding the structure of guidelines. The Latvian NHS is in charge of the application of the regulation.

Associations that are allowed to develop guidelines are regulated by Regulation No. 469; they are professional medical organizations (such as endocrinologists, cardiologists, pulmonologists, and so on), medical treatment institutions and institutions of higher education with academic study programmes in medicine.

The development of clinical guidelines per se is decentralized in Latvia; proposals for the development of clinical guidelines from the organizations have to be submitted to the NHS, along with a draft of the clinical guideline.

Quality control

According to Regulation No. 469, the NHS is responsible for assessing the quality of the clinical guidelines according to defined criteria, including the level of recommendation based on evidence-based medicine. The Centre of Health Economics (CHE) subsequently sends the draft to experts (the Board of Leading Specialists) at the Ministry of Health and to the Health Sector Council. If necessary, the CHE is able to send the project to other specialists/professional organizations.

The guidelines must fulfil the requirements stated in Regulation No. 469. Each treatment institution has a quality system in place, whereby treatment processes and the participation of medical personnel are controlled.

Professional associations also keep track of clinical guidelines, update them and submit new ones to the NHS according to Regulation No. 469.

Implementation

When the guidelines are approved they are registered by the NHS (which also notifies the Ministry of Health) and published on the NHS's home page (Latvian NHS, 2012), where they are publicly accessible. Their use is generally promoted through professional associations; it is planned that by the development of e-Health, their availability will improve.

Regulation No. 469 states that medical institutions shall implement the guidelines in compliance with their own financial possibilities.

Evaluation

The quality of health care is monitored by the Health Inspectorate. This is a national institution supervised by the Ministry of Health, which monitors and controls implementation of the binding laws and regulations affecting the health care sector. Its responsibilities are regulated by the Regulation of the Cabinet of Ministers No. 76 "Regulations of the Health Inspectorate" (adopted in 2008) (Latvian Health Inspectorate, 2008). Its framework also includes the control of medical treatment institutions, as well as the quality of professional health care services and of health care itself.

Lithuania

Background

Clinical guidelines exist in Lithuania for specific diseases (including diabetes, coronary heart disease, certain cancers, asthma, arthritis, and so on) and they are usually defined as "Diagnostics and treatment methodologies".

Regulatory basis

There is a legal basis for clinical guidelines development and implementation in Lithuania. The Order of the Minister of Health No. V-1148 (2008) provides the basic requirements for the development and implementation of diagnostics and treatment guidelines (Subata, 2009). Moreover, the Order of the Minister of Health No. V-338 (2008) defines that, in the absence of clinical guidelines approved by the Ministry of Health, the health institutions should prepare their own protocols to guarantee the quality of health service provision.

Development

Minister of Health Order No. V-1148 sets out methodological guidelines for clinical guideline development, including naming the possible initiators, evidence grading, the process of approval by the Ministry of Health, dissemination guidelines and implementation of the clinical guidelines.

Clinical guidelines can be developed by universities, research organizations, physicians' professional associations and/or Ministry of Health working groups. The regulations define the structure of the clinical guidelines and specify that they must present the Level of Evidence for given recommendations and the Class of the Recommendation (according to the standard evidence-based medicine levels).

Quality control

The development of clinical guidelines approved by the Ministry of Health involves close coordination with the Medical Faculties, National Health Insurance Fund, the State Pharmaceutical Control Service and the Mandatory Health Insurance Service.

Clinical guidelines developers are required to submit a draft of the clinical guidelines to be reviewed by two previously identified national universities and subsequently by specific agencies of the Ministry of Health. However, it is not mandatory for the final version of the clinical guidelines to be approved by the Ministry of Health; it can be used as a guiding document by professional associations or university clinics.

Implementation

Guidelines used are required to have been approved by the Ministry of Health. The Order of the Minister of Health No. V-338 (2008) relating to minimal standards in terms of the quality of health care services mandates health care institutions to follow the "Diagnostics and treatment methodologies" approved by the Ministry of Health.

The use of guidelines which have not been approved by the Ministry of Health, but which have been published in official sources (medical or research literature, web sites of universities, physicians' associations, health service providers' institutions and so on) are recommended for use in health care institutions for appropriate specialties. In the event that there are no national or local guidelines on specific conditions, it is recommended to follow WHO guidelines or the recommendations of international physicians' associations.

Evaluation

Development and quality control of clinical guidelines, as well as implementation and use of the guidelines, are evaluated through the audit processes, according to the legislation.

Luxembourg

Background

In Luxembourg, clinical guidelines only exist for a few conditions, for example for cardiovascular and cerebral diseases. The *Conseil Scientifique* plays a key role, consisting of members of the Ministry of Health, the medical examination services department of the social insurance system and various representatives of the associations of physicians and dentists. The web site of the *Conseil Scientifique* functions as an information platform and supports professionals and patients in their decision-making process (Conseil Scientifique, 2012).

Regulatory basis

Besides the *Conseil Scientifique*, no "official" basis for clinical guideline development and implementation exists as yet in Luxembourg. Various plans are being discussed, but no specific results are available.

Development

The development of clinical guidelines is centralized (undertaken by the *Conseil Scientifique* and the Ministry of Health). Different specialist groups submit proposals to put specific conditions or treatments on the agenda for guideline development, but this process is neither centralized nor coordinated.

Quality control

Clinical guidelines are not checked for quality before being implemented.

Implementation

The use of clinical guidelines is not mandatory. No information is available about incentive mechanisms and IT or other support tools.

Evaluation

The development, quality control, implementation and use of clinical guidelines are not evaluated.

Malta

Background

Clinical guidelines do exist in Malta; however, they focus more on acute conditions or acute exacerbations of chronic diseases, and none focus on the prevention or long-term management of chronic diseases. Moreover, their development and implementation are not regulated and are left instead to the initiative of clinicians.

Medicine protocols – used within the Government Health Services – are developed and implemented nationally by the Medicines Entitlement Unit and some of these cover medicines used in the treatment of chronic diseases.

The first national *Strategy for the Prevention and Control of Noncommunicable Disease* was published in 2010 by the Department of Health Promotion and Disease Prevention (2010) of the Ministry of Health, the Elderly and Community Care. It was an attempt by the Government to shift its focus from treatment and curative services to prevention services. The strategy identifies the development and implementation of national evidence-based guidelines on the primary and secondary prevention of NCDs as a priority for action.

Regulatory basis

No national body is charged with the task of developing and implementing clinical guidelines in Malta. Interested groups of clinicians have been developing clinical guidelines based on their own initiative(s).

Development

The development of clinical guidelines to be used at hospital level is left to clinicians working in Malta's main hospital (Mater Dei Hospital). The development process has been formalized and regulated through the CGCC in the Department of Medicine. Once a topic is identified, an independent GDG is established and the guideline is developed following the protocol developed by the SIGN. At Mater Dei Hospital, several interested departments are forming a group that will bring all the separate guideline development initiatives together in one portal. This is still in its initial stages and IT support is still being negotiated.

Only recently have clinical guidelines been developed in the primary care setting. Six clinical guidelines – mostly related to the acute management of pre-hospital medical emergencies – have been developed, by adapting international clinical guidelines, through a collaborative process between a lead practitioner in Family Medicine and relevant specialists from Mater Dei Hospital.

Quality control

Review processes do exist for clinical guidelines developed at secondary and primary care levels; however, no specific instruments are used to validate them.

Clinical guidelines developed by hospital clinicians undergo an internal review process. The draft must be approved by the CGCC and the legal department of the hospital, in order to be approved and disseminated. For clinical guidelines developed in the primary care setting a draft version circulates among stakeholders for feedback and amendments. The final document must be authorized by the Director of Primary Health.

There is no formal procedure for updating the guidelines and this is normally carried out when the related international guideline is updated.

Implementation

No formal processes exist for the implementation of clinical guidelines in Malta and their use is not mandatory. Clinical guidelines in use at Mater Dei Hospital are available in hard copy (paper format), but also electronically, through the hospital intranet. The primary care guidelines are endorsed by the Primary Health Department and these are simply disseminated to health centres in hard copy.

Evaluation

No formal evaluation of clinical guidelines takes place in Malta.

In hospitals the guidelines are periodically evaluated by the CGCC. In the primary care setting, no audit has yet been performed but plans are under way for this to take place in the near future.

The Netherlands

Background

The Netherlands have significant experience in the field of guidelines. Clinical guidelines do exist in primary and specialist care, specifically relating to preventing and treating chronic diseases. A multitude of other tools support professionals and chronically ill patients in their decision-making: information from organizations and consultants, continuing education, decision support software, virtual networks, and so on.

Regulatory basis

There is no official basis for the development and implementation of clinical guidelines in the Netherlands. Different organizations produce clinical guidelines, such as the RIVM (RIVM, 2012), the CBO (CBO, 2012), the Dutch Council for Quality of Care, as well as the NHG (NHG, 2012). Clinical guidelines are also introduced indirectly by the development and implementation of Disease Management Programmes.

Development

As already mentioned, clinical guidelines production is carried out at a centralized level. Additionally, in primary care, the NHG plays a key role in the development of clinical guidelines. Since almost all Dutch general practitioners are members of the NHG, clinical guideline development can be considered to be centralized by this institution. The Dutch Council for Quality of Care (Regieraad) conducts research and development, implementation and updating of guidelines, and works on the harmonization of guideline development in the Netherlands (Regieraad Kwaliteit van Zorg, 2012). Other organizations involved in the development of clinical guidelines include: the Dutch Association of Comprehensive Cancer Centres, the Netherlands Institute of Mental Health & Addiction (Trimbos), the Royal Dutch Society for Physical Therapy (KNGF) (KNGF, 2012), and the Netherlands Centre for Excellence in Nursing (LEVV). Furthermore, in 1997 a national IT platform (EBRO) was initiated by the Dutch Cochrane Centre and the Dutch Institute for Healthcare Improvement to support the clinical guideline development process and use of clinical guidelines (G-I-N, 2010). Most of these organizations publish the clinical guidelines on their web sites.

Quality control

There is no published evidence on quality control ahead of implementation. Methods used differ among organizations: for example, while the NHG uses the nominal group technique to check clinical guidelines before implementation, other groups use piloting as their method of choice.

Implementation

The use of clinical guidelines in the Dutch health care system is obligatory only in certain cases, for example in end-of-life care. To support the implementation and application of clinical guidelines by professionals, different insurers provide financial incentives. Legislation on quality of health care organizations or patient–doctor interactions indirectly influences the utilization of clinical guidelines on behalf of practitioners.

Evaluation

There is no official regulation underpinning the evaluation of clinical guidelines. Individual research projects by scientific researchers, insurers or professionals evaluate (methods of) quality control. In terms of implementation, there is still a lack of evaluation. However, several studies have been published to evaluate the implementation and impact of clinical guidelines (Burgers & Van Everdingen, 2004; Frijling et al., 2002; Van Bruggen et al., 2008; Verstappen et al., 2003; Lub et al., 2006).

Norway

Background

Clinical guidelines exist in Norway on both prevention and treatment of chronic diseases; some clinical guidelines focus specifically on prevention or treatment, but most deal with prevention, diagnostics and treatment.

Regulatory basis

The "official" basis for clinical guideline development and implementation is the Norwegian Directorate of Health. The Directorate is the only institution with a mandate to develop national clinical guidelines. The Directorate is both responsible for and "owns" the guidelines, but often works on behalf of the Ministry of Health and Care Services, and the guidelines are usually developed in close cooperation with representatives from relevant specialist groups and other key stakeholders, such as the Norwegian Medicines Agency and patient interests groups.

Development

Official national clinical guidelines are developed centrally, as already described. The Directorate of Health is also responsible for the development of "priority guidelines" in cooperation with Norway's four Regional Health Authorities. The priority guidelines are developed to give support to the specialists involved in deciding priority levels when dealing with referrals to hospitals. Other guidelines are developed in a decentralized manner, often by the Medical Societies of the Norwegian Medical Association; one example is the "guideline on diabetes, pre-diabetes and cardiovascular disease", developed by the Norwegian Society of Cardiology. The Norwegian Board of Health Supervision has developed, on behalf of the Directorate of Health, a "guideline for developing clinical guideline guidelines" in cooperation with the Norwegian Medical Association, among others. The Directorate has also compiled a "reference book on developing clinical guidelines" in cooperation with the Norwegian Electronic Health Library and the Norwegian Knowledge Centre for the Health Services.

The need to revise a national clinical guideline is expected to be considered within three years of publication of the guideline.

Quality control

A draft of the national clinical guideline is required to be sent for both internal and external evaluation/consultation. In the development of certain national clinical guidelines, an external "reference group" is also established to evaluate the process.

Clinical guidelines are checked for quality using the AGREE instrument before being implemented. The instrument is used both during the development process and before implementation by the Secretariat of the Directorate of Health (requirement) and by the Norwegian Electronic Health Library before publishing the guideline online.

Implementation

The use of national guidelines is not mandatory in Norway. The "Priority

Guidelines" describe the Norwegian Health Authorities' view on the right interpretation of the current legislature, but are not considered as "binding" documents for health service providers. No financial incentives exist for the implementation and use of national clinical guidelines. The use of clinical guidelines is promoted through web sites, some developed with interactive learning. Certain guidelines related to practical clinical implementation are integrated as IT applications in electronic patient record systems.

Evaluation

No data were available on evaluation of the implementation of clinical guidelines.

Poland

Background

Clinical guidelines exist in Poland, both for chronic conditions (such as COPD, asthma, hypertension and diabetes) and acute conditions (such as pulmonary embolism and deep vein thrombosis (DVT)). The National Pharmaceutical Policy for 2004–2008 published in 2003 identified a need for the development of ambulatory health care formularies (*receptariusz lecznictwa ambulatoryjnego*), which would contain guidelines on the use of medications in specific cases and set standards of medical treatment, taking into account their costs. Work on these formularies is still in progress.

Regulatory basis

A national standard or legal basis for clinical guidelines development does not yet exist.

Development

The development of clinical guidelines is decentralized. Given the lack of a legal basis for clinical guideline development, different institutions can be involved in the clinical guidelines development process, for example professional organizations, specialists, medical societies or the CoPFiP. The process is not coordinated and no guidance on standardizing clinical guidelines development exists.

Quality control

No requirement exists to perform a quality check on clinical guidelines before their implementation. The CoPFiP uses the Delphi approach for consensus among the panel of experts and practitioners involved. Some existing clinical guidelines already include quality instruments, such as the clinical guidelines for DVT or pulmonary embolism.

Implementation

Clinical guidelines are not binding in Poland. Furthermore, no incentives exist to implement and use established guidelines. To promote the application of clinical guidelines by general practitioners, workshops, seminars, lectures and publications in *Lekarz Rodzinny*[13] have been carried out by theCoPFiP.

Evaluation

The evaluation of clinical guidelines is not mandatory and is only carried out to a limited extent. The CoPFiP partially monitors the implementation of clinical guidelines and sporadic research projects have been initiated on the utilization of clinical guidelines.

Portugal

Background

In Portugal, clinical guidelines exist on preventing and treating chronic diseases, as well as for other conditions. The trend towards development and implementation of clinical guidelines is being fast-tracked due to the current financial crisis, and as one of the measures in the Troika's "Memorandum of understanding". The Memorandum states that Portugal should continue with the publication of clinical guidelines and put in place a system to audit their implementation.

Regulatory basis

As a government body, the DGS has the legal duty of producing and implementing guidelines. They are developed and implemented as part of government documents, NSFs, within Disease Management Programmes, as well as through guidance produced by quasi-official agencies. In addition to the DGS, several medical societies for sub-specialties and the APMGF also develop clinical guidelines.

---

13 Polish journal entitled *Family Physician*.

Development

Given that the main responsibility for clinical guidelines lies with the DGS, the development process is carried out centrally. In June 2011, the DGS started a new method for designing guidelines in a joint project with the Portuguese Medical Association (*Ordem dos Médicos*), the colleges, and the medical societies, including the APMGF; 70 guidelines have been produced and are currently the subject of public discussion. The final versions will be subject to an evaluation before being approved by a body of experts, the Scientific Committee for Good Clinical Practice, which includes several general practitioner academics.

Quality control

There is no formal requirement for checking the quality of clinical guidelines before implementation, and this is therefore not undertaken.

Implementation

When the new framework is approved, the use of clinical guidelines will be mandatory for all physicians working in Portugal, both in the public and private sectors. Currently, to support the implementation and use of clinical guidelines, financial incentives exist for doctors, nurses and staff, based on their score in the annual audit of family physician performance (obligatory for family physicians under the new regulation). Furthermore, the implementation and use of clinical guidelines are promoted through various disease-specific IT tools (in place for diabetes (Barahona et al., 2001), hypertension, cancer screening, child care, maternal care and family planning), as well as web sites (such as the DGS web site (DGS, 2012)) and accompanying specialized literature.

Evaluation

No evidence is available on the evaluation of the development, implementation and use of clinical guidelines. According to various experts, evaluation is carried out from within the DGS, along with agencies and bodies that issue guidelines. No publications exist on clinical guideline evaluation. However, the performance indicators used in the annual audit of family physician performance are being reviewed by the ACSS.

Romania

Background

Clinical guidelines exist in Romania in general terms, and for chronic conditions in particular, such as for type 2 diabetes mellitus, low lumbar pain, depression, asthma and malignancies.

Regulatory basis

The development of clinical guidelines is the responsibility of the Ministry of Health. The actual task is delegated to expert groups from different clinical specialties, officially appointed by the Ministry to provide advice and guidance in their respective fields. A Governmental Decision (HG 351/2012) was published on 24 April 2012 to modify the structure of the Ministry of Health to include an HTA department. Among other tass, the new HTA department will be responsible for the development of methodological guidelines for HTA and development of clinical guidelines in close collaboration with other institutions.

Clinical guidelines are described by several legal documents that are currently in effect (government programmes, Ministry of Health orders, and so on).

Development

The Ministry of Health has appointed 10 special "commissions" for different medical fields (such as the Commission for Oncology), which consist of experts and develop recommendations in their specialties. These are ALBs that have used not only specifications provided in the Ministerial Order establishing them, but also existing international guidance to form recommendations. Special attention was paid to consensus processes.

No explicit methodology exists for the development of clinical guidelines.

Clinical guidelines are also developed by the National Centre for Family Medicine, aimed at family doctors. These are endorsed by the National Society for Family Medicine and are not connected to governmental mandates. The National Centre for Family Medicine has produced a methodology for developing clinical guidelines for its own guidance (CNSMF, 2012).

Quality control

There is no indication that the quality of clinical guidelines is monitored before implementation. However, for the 10 practice guidelines produced by the Commissions, as described in the previous subsection, the AGREE instrument was used before finalizing the guideline to ensure due process had been followed.

Implementation

Clinicians are expected to implement the clinical guidelines developed by the Ministry of Health. However, the publication of a clinical guideline is not associated with a particular process of implementation, and no monitoring mechanisms exist to evaluate practitioner compliance. Clinical guidelines developed by the National Centre for Family Medicine are endorsed by the National Society for Family Medicine, but they are not compulsory. While clinical guidelines are available online, there are no user-friendly IT applications aimed at facilitating their utilization.

Financial incentives are in place and are operationalized by means of a provider's contract with the insurance fund. Health units that have developed and implement treatment protocols based on national guidelines receive additional funding. While IT applications are not yet widespread to support the implementation of clinical guidelines, both press conferences and publications have been organized to ensure awareness.

Evaluation

There is no indication of the existence or type of evaluation after the publication of a clinical guideline. Since the process of clinical guideline production in Romania is still at an early stage, it is expected that related mechanisms will be developed in the future.

Slovakia

Background

There is currently no official basis for the development of clinical guidelines on chronic conditions in Slovakia. The few existing guidelines that are up to date have been developed by specialist medical associations (for example, for cardiology) and usually consist of translated European recommendations. Slovakian physicians often refer to guidance produced by the Czech National College of General Practice, when Slovakian recommendations on a given condition are not available.

Regulatory basis

A clear regulatory basis on clinical guidelines is currently lacking in Slovakia.

Development

There is both centralized and decentralized guidance production, although not coordinated in a comprehensive way. The Institute of Preventive Medicine, with the support of the Slovakian Ministry of Health, was active in the field of clinical guidelines some years ago, producing the handbooks for diagnostic and therapeutic guidelines, including the most important and frequent chronic conditions. Unfortunately, these were last updated in 2002 and no longer reflect current practice. Since 2001, single guidelines are being developed by the Central Commission of Rational Pharmacotherapy and Drug Policy of the Ministry of Health. Between 2000 and 2002 these were published regularly, but since then only sporadically. They do not cover the most important chronic conditions and practitioners often use international recommendations to aid their decision-making process. In 2004 the National Institute of Quality and Innovations (NIKI) (NIKI, 2005b) was established, aiming to develop and implement national clinical guidelines. Upon establishment, the NIKI published a handbook (NIKI, 2005a) for developing national clinical guidelines but has not produced specific guidance since then. It is therefore unclear to what extent the handbook is in use but it is in any case not mandatory. Given the deregulation of contracting in the Slovakian health system, health insurance companies have experimented with the introduction of formal clinical guidelines for chronic conditions, but so far all initiatives have failed in the quality control implementation phase.

Quality control

Given that the production of clinical guidelines is not officially supervised or coordinated, no claim for quality control can be made.

Implementation

Guidance utilization is not mandatory. This is, however, an issue that is on the agenda of the Ministry of Health.

Evaluation

No official evaluation mechanism for clinical guidelines is currently in place.

Slovenia

Background

Slovenia does not have a comprehensive suite of clinical guidelines. Moreover, they are poorly implemented and their implementation is inadequately assessed.

International guidance is used in many of the services that are delivered, but currently only on an ad hoc basis. A wide range of various guidelines and recommendations are published in the *Slovene Medical Journal* and several other journals; however, the methodology behind the reviewed guideline development is rarely stated. As no national body is responsible for the clinical guidelines, they are mainly developed by groups of experts.

Regulatory basis

There is no legal framework or official basis for clinical guideline development and implementation in Slovenia. However, in 2003 the Ministry of Health published guidance on the development of clinical practice guidelines (Slovenian Ministry of Health, 2003).

The proposal for the Health Services Act of 2010 envisioned an Agency for Quality and Safety that would have been in charge of clinical guidelines. However, this proposal was abolished by the current Minister of Health, and a new proposal is currently being prepared. According to a personal communication, the Agency is still forecast within the new proposal. In addition to the tasks of setting standards for quality and safety indicators, introducing clinical pathways and so on, the agency will also have the task of authorizing and implementing clinical guidelines.

Development

Development of clinical guidelines is the domain of experts; mainly medical associations for various specialties. The Slovene *Manual on development of clinical practice guidelines* (Slovenian Ministry of Health, 2003) takes into account some traditional models of programmes for the preparation of guidelines, such as the SIGN (2012), the ÄZQ (2010) and the G-I-N (2012). However, the manual is often not used in developing guidelines; they are mainly developed based upon the consensus of the experts in a certain field. Nevertheless, some clinical guidelines (such as those for diabetes) explicitly state the level of evidence used for the guidelines.

Quality control

According to the aforementioned *Manual on development of clinical practice guidelines*, the AGREE tool should be used for quality control; however, as use of the manual is not mandatory for clinical guideline development, there is currently no quality control or any kind of evaluation of clinical guidelines.

The forecast Agency for Quality and Safety would be in charge of evaluating the quality and implementation of clinical guidelines.

Implementation

Clinical guidelines are not mandatory in Slovenia; they are considered to be a support tool for health workers in their decision-making processes.

Currently, no explicit discussion is under way on how to drive and control the implementation of clinical guidelines at national level; it is expected that the Agency for Quality and Safety will be responsible for implementation and quality control of future guidelines.

Evaluation

The development, quality control, implementation and use of clinical guidelines have not been regularly evaluated so far.

Spain

Background

The Spanish National Health System Quality Agency of the Ministry of Health, through a national programme for the development of clinical guidelines (coordinated by GuíaSalud) centralizes the elaboration and publication of clinical guidelines in Spain. A total of 35 clinical guidelines are currently available from this National Programme, ranging from treatment to prevention and from specific to generic diseases. However, their implementation varies. Moreover, competences in health policies are currently transferred to the regional governments (the Autonomous Communities), which makes the clinical guidelines implementation situation particularly heterogeneous across the regions. Some of the HTA agencies and units are active agents in the promotion of clinical guidelines and standards.

Regulatory basis

The Spanish Ministry of Health developed (in 2006) a Quality Plan for the

National Health System that includes the strategy of "Improving clinical excellence" and specific objectives related to clinical guidelines. In terms of policy, the use of clinical guidelines is not mandatory in Spain. Incentives depend on the regulatory framework of each Autonomous Community (region).

Development

The Spanish National Health System Quality Agency of the Ministry of Health (GuíaSalud) commissions the process of elaboration and publication, establishing agreements with the different HTA agencies and units responsible for developing the clinical guideline in each case. Clinical guidelines are funded through these agreements, and the amount of funds is negotiated on a case-by-case basis. This coordination also involves solving possible problems of concurrence between the agents participating in the process. The first agreement was reached in 2006 and it has been extended annually or biannually until 2011. The entity responsible for developing the clinical guidelines provides the working group and selects the external reviewers, although GuíaSalud provides a list of proposed participants from which to choose. The scientific societies and the patients' associations relevant to the clinical condition of the specific clinical guideline are always among the agents consulted. Other stakeholders involved in the development may include: clinical leaders; other clinical experts, such as nurses or pharmacists; experts in the development of clinical guidelines; librarians; patients'/carers' associations; technical coordinators; and other experts (epidemiologists, health economists, lawyers, qualitative technicians, experts in statistics, and so on).

Methodological experts (experts in the elaboration of clinical guidelines) are usually responsible for systematic reviews, although this depends on each working group. Consensus is usually informally reached within the working group involved in elaborating the clinical guideline. HTA agencies and units (regions) could also promote and individually fund the development of a clinical guideline, although incentives for coordination do exist, in so far as coordination is a requirement from the Spanish Ministry of Health in order to allocate funds to a guideline. There is still no *ex ante* process to decide a list of guidelines to be elaborated and funded by the Clinical Practice Guideline Programme, and coordination is achieved by initiating a call for submissions, in which various key people participate, proposing individual topics for consideration.

Currently, the Clinical Practice Guideline Programme (GuíaSalud) is working on methodological handbooks for the development of clinical guidelines, with the aim of facilitating the participation of patients (GuíaSalud, 2012c).

Quality control

Quality control measures include the use of the AGREE tool and external reviews, including a public consultation period. Such measures are not mandatory, but are the standard procedure before publishing and using a clinical guideline. The quality control system remains prominent in the Clinical Practice Guideline Programme's agenda for ensuring the implementation and use of clinical guidelines.

Implementation

In Spain, the implementation of guidelines in health care is not mandatory and the decision lies with the Autonomous Communities (regional level). No specific incentives exist to implement clinical guidelines at national level, although the Autonomous Communities can introduce these incentives through purchase agreements with providers – partially linked to quality results – or can make the use of guidelines mandatory in publicly run centres.

Clinical guidelines are still not particularly well implemented in Spain. Nevertheless, the Clinical Practice Guideline Programme of the Spanish National Health System (GuíaSalud) includes three methodological handbooks to cover users' needs in each of the three stages of the development of the clinical guideline, and one of them relates to implementation. It sets out some recommendations and specifies which strategies for implementation have been proven to be most effective. Each Autonomous Community is responsible for implementation, resulting in a particularly heterogeneous implementation situation. It seems that, in most cases, implementation is a matter of trust and depends on the degree of participation in the elaboration process. So (since the use of clinical guidelines not mandatory), professionals tend to implement the guidelines developed by the HTA agencies and units of their own Autonomous Communities (regions). Regional ministries of health from the different Autonomous Communities are going to take part in the GuíaSalud Consultant Committee, and this is likely to serve as a platform to promote implementation.

Evaluation

No formal evaluation takes place at any stage of the process (development, quality control or implementation). However, as mentioned in the previous subsections, the Clinical Practice Guidelines Programme of the Spanish National Health System (GuíaSalud) includes three methodological handbooks on the development stages of the guideline: development, updating and implementation. The development, implementation and use of guidelines have changed dramatically since the early 2000s in Spain. The quality of the clinical guidelines has improved a great deal, since the aforementioned development handbook was published and quality control measures (such as the AGREE tool) have been widely implemented. Progress regarding implementation and evaluation of clinical guidelines are now among the priorities of the Clinical Practice Guideline Programme within the Spanish National Health System (GuíaSalud).

Sweden

Background

In Sweden, clinical guidelines exist both for chronic diseases and NCDs (such as diabetes, renal failure, coronary heart disease, cataract surgery, stroke, hip fracture and hip replacement, as well as malignant neoplasms) (Nolte, Knai & McKee, 2008). Other initiatives to enhance care for chronic conditions – such as the establishment of disease-specific nurse-led clinics – are also in place.

Regulatory basis

The responsibility for developing clinical guidelines lies primarily with the NBHW, an agency under the Ministry of Health and Social Affairs. However, given the structure of the Swedish health care system, counties and municipalities – which also have a degree of autonomy – also develop clinical guidelines, even though regional and local clinical guidelines are often based on national guidelines.[14]

Development

The development of clinical guidelines is predominantly centralized and carried out by the NBHW. Apart from the NBHW, the Swedish Association of Local Authorities and Regions (SALAR), as well as the Swedish Council on Technology Assessment in Health Care (SBU) are integrated in the development process. The participation of the SALAR in the clinical guidelines development process is intended to bring about better consideration of regional interests in terms of topic choice and organizational and financial impact. However, some Swedish counties and municipalities still develop their own clinical guidelines. The SBU provides guidance on methodological issues, particularly in regard to evidence retrieval and synthesis.

The NBHW is in charge of selecting guidelines to be developed and providing guidance on their development. The clinical guidelines to be developed are chosen according to the burden of disease in the country, the cost of the specific

---

14 More information is available at the web site of the NBHW (Socialstyrelsen, 2012).

disease and to what extent there has been demand for guidance on the part of decision-makers and the professions concerned. Once the NBHW has chosen a guideline to be developed, a pool of experts (called the Fact Group) is selected to work on it. The Fact Group should perform a systematic review of the evidence, first using information from the SBU and the NBHW, and subsequently from other sources. In the meantime, a CEA of the intervention is carried out by a pool of experts in health economics. Afterwards, a "prioritizing" group (consisting of experts with strong backgrounds in health and medical care) ranks the intervention according to the severity of the condition, the strength of the scientific evidence on the effect of the intervention and its cost–effectiveness. The ranking is important for supporting the subsequent decision-making on the distribution of resources. Next, a preliminary version of the guideline is compiled, as well as a shorter version for the lay public. The final version of the guideline is later published on the NBHW web site (Socialstyrelsen, 2011). The guidelines also include recommendations on measures that should not be implemented at all ("Do Not Do" measures), whereby those particular measures have no effect or may entail risks for the patient.

Quality control

Little is known about quality control before implementation. Evidence is available confirming that quality assessment procedures are carried out, but not which quality system/instrument is applied.

Implementation

The use of guidelines is endorsed but no penalties are in place for non-compliance. Several tools to facilitate the implementation and use of clinical guidelines exist, such as publications, educational materials, conferences, IT applications, and so on. Moreover, updated clinical guidelines are sent to each registered practitioner. In some areas, financial incentives also exist.

Evaluation

The final version of the clinical guidelines should also include indicators of a good standard of care that can be used to track the improvement in health care after the guidelines have been implemented, as well as their impact. The development, quality control, implementation and use of clinical guidelines are regularly evaluated by the NBHW, as well as by county councils or universities (on request) (Socialstyrelsen, 2011).

Switzerland

Background

In Switzerland, recommendations for best practice exist on the prevention and treatment of chronic conditions (for example, hyperlipidaemia, asthma and hypertension), as well as for other clinical conditions. These mostly stem from professional organizations or are international standards adapted to the Swiss context and reviewed by a group of experts. There are no centrally or largely distributed tools to assist professionals and patients in their decision-making. Most related initiatives are implemented on a local basis and their dissemination is therefore limited.

Regulatory basis

There is no formal legislation and therefore no official basis for the development of clinical guidelines; and no agencies exist that are formally mandated with the development of clinical guidelines in Switzerland. National societies and associations mostly lag behind existing best practice recommendations and both institutional and financial support for the development of decision-making aids is limited. Initiatives in the realm of disease management are still in their infancy and the related regulatory framework is lacking. However, several local and small initiatives are under way in several cantons. For example, in the French-speaking Vaud canton, a programme on the prevention and management of diabetes was launched in 2010 and a series of related clinical guidelines are currently being developed.

Development

Guidelines are developed either by professional associations or foundations or, even more locally, by small groups of physicians. These clinical guidelines quite often comprise an adaptation of international guidelines to the local context. Some have been published in local papers. No general guidelines exist for clinical guideline development.

Quality control

There is no recent evaluation of the number, origin or quality of clinical guidelines produced. The AGREE and ADAPTE instruments are used by certain hubs, such as the one at the University of Lausanne. However, there is no information as to the extent to which guideline production, adaptation or implementation is based on best evidence.

Implementation

The use of clinical guidelines is not mandatory and there are no financial incentives encouraging their use. Practitioners are completely free to decide whether or how they are going to use the guidelines. Local directives regarding medical services in certain hospitals may be the exception to this rule. As IT developments in the health sector are still in their infancy in Switzerland, there is no nationwide IT-based implementation of guidelines. However, local initiatives do exist, particularly in terms of electronic medical records. They are not implemented in all hospitals, but rather only sporadically in ambulatory care. There is no information on the extent to which clinical guidelines are actually being used in Swiss health care provision.

Evaluation

There is no formal evaluation of the development, quality, implementation and use of clinical guidelines in Switzerland. It is safe to assume that professional organizations or local clinical guideline developers update their recommendations, but there is no related coordination or supervision.

United Kingdom (England)

Background

In England, clinical guidelines exist for the management and prevention of several conditions, both chronic and otherwise (for example, for the prevention of myocardial infarction: secondary prevention, obesity, alcohol-use disorders, type 2 diabetes mellitus, CVD, mental health and behavioural conditions, and so on). All the clinical guidelines are published and accessible via the NICE web site (NICE, 2012a).

The NICE is the independent organization responsible for providing national guidance and setting quality standards relating to the promotion of good health and the prevention and treatment of ill health. The NICE produces guidance on public health, health technologies (pharmaceuticals, interventional procedures, devices and diagnostics) and clinical practice. It makes recommendations to the NHS, local authorities and other organizations in the public, private and voluntary sectors on new and existing medicines, treatments and procedures and on treating and caring for people with specific diseases and conditions.

All the recommendations, standards and services are developed by the NICE in consultation with independent committees and experts working in health care, academia and industry, alongside patients and members of the public with a background or interest in the area. The NCCCC – which is funded by the NICE and based at the RCP – leads on developing clinical guidelines for the treatment of chronic conditions. The Centre for Public Health Excellence provides guidance on services that contribute to the prevention of chronic conditions and encourage good health and well-being.

Regulatory basis

The NICE was set up in 1999 to ensure equal access to medical treatments and high-quality care from the NHS across England and Wales. The Department of Health commissions the NICE to develop clinical guidelines, guidance on public health and technology appraisals.

Health care professionals are expected to take NICE clinical guidelines fully into account when exercising their clinical judgement. However, the guidance does not override the responsibility of health care professionals to make decisions appropriate to the circumstances of each patient. These decisions should be made in consultation with, and with the agreement of, the patient and/or their guardian or carer. Health care professionals are expected to record their reasons for not following clinical guideline recommendations.

Development

In England, clinical guidelines are developed centrally through the NICE, NCCs (funded by the NICE) and the Royal Colleges, but may be adapted and implemented at the local level through NHS Hospital Trusts, PCTs, local authorities and voluntary organizations.

Guideline topics are usually referred by the Department of Health and health care professionals when there is confusion or uncertainty about the value of a drug, device, treatment or interventional procedure. Topics are prioritized on the basis of the related burden of disease, resource impact of the proposed guideline, importance in relation to government policy and the level of variation in clinical practice.

Various stakeholders – such as national patient and carer organizations, health care professionals, academics, industry representatives, service providers and commissioners – register their interest and are consulted throughout the process. The NCC commissioned to develop the guideline prepares the scope and sets out what the guideline will and will not cover. An independent GDG is established and members are recruited through formal adverts on the NICE web site, followed by an application and interview process. Members are required to undergo formal training on the guideline development process.

Any conflict of interest must be declared by members when applying to join the group and at the beginning of every meeting, in case their status changes.

The group considers the evidence and reaches conclusions based on this. In cases in which evidence is poor or lacking, a process of informal expert consensus is used to make decisions. Exceptionally, if the literature search has found no evidence that addresses the review question, the group may identify best practice by using formal consensus methods outside the GDG (for example, the Delphi technique or the nominal group technique).

There is at least one public consultation period lasting eight weeks, during which registered stakeholders can comment on the draft guideline. At this time the NICE commissions expert peer reviewers to carry out a statistical and health economics review. The GDG takes into consideration all the input from the consultation and makes the appropriate changes to the guideline.

An independent guideline review panel validates the guideline, paying particular attention to how the GDG addressed comments received during the consultation. The panel must also make sure that it will be feasible for the NHS to implement the final recommendations. The NICE Guidance Executive approves the final version of the guideline before it is published.

Guidelines are normally considered for an update three years after publication, but partial updates may be carried out earlier than this if significant new evidence emerges.

Quality control

The guideline development process is based on the AGREE instrument (AGREE Collaboration, 2001) and described in a comprehensive manner in *The guidelines manual 2009* (NICE, 2009b). The stakeholder consultation, expert reviews and the assessment by the independent guideline review panel are all part of the validation process. Prior to publication, the guidelines are subjected to an internal quality control assessment at the Centre for Clinical Practice. NHS Evidence assesses guidance producers for quality in order to allow users to recognize sources of information of the highest quality, awarding them with a seal of approval in the form of an Accreditation Mark.

Guidelines are not piloted but are developed in a collaborative process with practitioners and service users. As mentioned, the independent guideline review panel also has a role in making sure that it will be feasible for the NHS to implement the final recommendations.

The ultimate test of the validity of NICE Guidelines took place during a judicial review in 2009. A claim against the NICE was brought by two CFS/

ME patients. The grounds of the challenge included an allegation of bias against the GDG and its members, that the guideline was irrational compared to the evidence, and claims relating to the classification of the condition and treatments recommended. The High Court ruled in favour of the NICE on all grounds brought against it (NICE, 2009a).

Implementation

Clinical guidelines are advisory rather than compulsory, but should be taken into account by health care professionals when planning care for individual patients. All NHS organizations are expected to meet NICE standards to ensure that everyone receives the same high-quality care.

The NICE supports the implementation of its guidance by engaging stakeholders that are encouraged to use their networks and influence to support implementation of the guidelines at national and local levels. The NICE has a team of implementation consultants that work nationally to encourage a supportive environment, as well as locally to share learning and support education and training. Generic implementation tools are available, such as a *"How to"* guide, along with specific tools for every clinical guideline, such as a costing template that can be used to estimate the local costs and savings involved in implementation, a PowerPoint presentation that highlights the key priorities and provides a framework for local discussion, and support for clinical auditing to help monitor and review local practice. Other tools which may be produced jointly with organizations such as professional or patient groups can include implementation advice to aid with action planning at an organizational level, referral letter templates, flow charts, fact sheets and checklists. The NICE works with universities and the Royal Colleges to help future and current NHS staff understand their role and it has proposed a set of initiatives to support future and current NHS staff in their education and professional development.

Shared learning: implementing NICE guidance (NICE, 2012c) is a quality-assured resource, freely available through the NICE web site, whereby practitioners share their innovative and successful approaches to implementing the guidance.

The development of NICE Quality Standards (to which the NHS must adhere) has become an important lever in supporting the implementation of the guidelines. For example, through the new Department of Health Commissioning for Quality and Innovation framework, a hospital could stand to lose 0.3% of its income if it fails to screen 90% of its patients for DVT.

Evaluation

The NICE produces implementation reports which measure the uptake of specific recommendations taken from selected pieces of guidance through the analysis of routine data. Interested researchers assess the uptake and effectiveness of guidance on an ad hoc basis. For example, a paper published in the *British Medical Journal* (Thornhill et al., 2011) showed that, despite a 78.6% reduction in prescribing of antibiotic prophylaxis after the introduction of the related NICE Guideline, the study excluded any large increase in the incidence of cases of (or deaths from) infective endocarditis in the two years after the guideline was implemented. Both kinds of reports are collated by the NICE in a central searchable database (NICE, 2010).

References

Aakre KM et al. (2010). Diagnosing microalbuminuria and consequences for the drug treatment of patients with type 2 diabetes: a European survey in primary care. *Diabetes Research and Clinical Practice*, 89(2):103–109.

AFSSAPS (2012). Agence nationale de sécurité du médicament et des produits de santé [web site]. Saint Denis, French Agency for the Safety of Health Products (ANSM) (http://www.afssaps.fr/, accessed 15 September 2012).

AGENAS (2012a). L'agenzia [The agency] [web site]. Rome, Italian National Agency for Regional Healthcare Systems (http://www.agenas.it/agenzia.html, accessed 20 August 2012).

AGENAS (2012b). L'Agenzia nazionale per i servizi sanitari regionali [National Agency for Regional Healthcare Systems] [web site]. Rome, Italian National Agency for Regional Healthcare Systems (http://www.agenas.it/index.htm, accessed 15 September 2012).

AGREE Collaboration (2001). *The appraisal of guidelines for research & evaluation (AGREE) instrument, 2001*. London, Agree Research Trust (http://www.agreetrust.org/resource-centre/, accessed 20 August 2012).

AGREE Collaboration (2003). Development and validation of an international appraisal instrument for assessing the quality of clinical practice guidelines: the AGREE project. *Quality and Safety in Health Care*, 12(1):18–23.

AGREE Collaboration (2010). Resource centre [web site]. Hamilton, ON, AGREE Collaboration (http://www.agreetrust.org/resource-centre/, accessed 20 August 2012).

AkdÄ (2012). Arzneimittelkommission der deutschen Ärzteschaft [web site]. Berlin, Arzneimittelkommission der deutschen Ärzteschaft (http://www.akdae.de/en/index.html, accessed 15 September 2012).

Alkin A (2001). Medizinische Leitlinien – Informationen für die ärztliche Praxis. *Guidelines*, 2:62–68.

Alonso-Coello P et al. (2008). Quality of guidelines on obesity in children is worrying. *British Medical Journal*, 337:a2474.

Alonso-Coello P et al. (2010). The quality of clinical practice guidelines over the last two decades: a systematic review of guideline appraisal studies. *Quality and Safety in Health Care*, 19(6):e58.

ANSM (2012). Agence nationale de sécurité du médicament et des produits de santé [web site]. Saint Denis, National Security Agency of Medicines and Health Products (http://ansm.sante.fr/?UserSpace=default, accessed 20 August 2012).

AQUA Institute (2012a). Cross-sectoral quality in health care [web site]. Göttingen, Institute for Applied Quality Assurance and Research in Healthcare (AQUA) (http://www.sqg.de/startseite/index-en.html, accessed 15 September 2012).

AQUA Institute (2012b). Zukunft durch Qualität. Innovative Lösungen und praxisnahe Konzepte für eine optimierte Gesundheitsversorgung [web site]. Göttingen, Institute for Applied Quality Assurance and Research in Healthcare (AQUA) (http://www.aqua-institut.de/de/home/index.html, accessed 15 September 2012).

Arznei & Vernunft (2012). Initiative Arznei & Vernunft ['Medicine & common sense' initiative] [web site]. Vienna, Arznei & Vernunft (http://www.arzneiundvernunft.info/content/index.php, accessed 20 August 2012).

Asmar R (2007). A specific training on hypertension guidelines improves blood pressure control by more than 10% in hypertensive patients: the VALNORM study. *Journal of the American Society of Hypertension*, 1(4):278–285.

Audet AM, Greenfield S, Field M (1990). Medical practice guidelines: current activities and future directions. *Annals of Internal Medicine*, 113(9):709–714.

Austrian Federal Health Commission (2010). *Quality strategy for the Austrian health care system*. Vienna, Austrian Federal Health Commission.

AWMF (2012a). Leitlinien [web site]. Düsseldorf, Association of the Scientific Medical Societies (AWMF) (http://www.awmf.org/leitlinien/aktuelle-leitlinien.html, accessed 20 August 2012).

AWMF (2012b). Leitlinien-Suche [online database]. Düsseldorf, Association of the Scientific Medical Societies (AWMF) (http://www.awmf.org/leitlinien/leitlinien-suche.html, accessed 30 September 2011).

AWMF, ÄZQ (2000). Leitlinien-Manual [web site]. Düsseldorf, Association of the Scientific Medical Societies (AWMF) and the German Agency for Quality in Medicine (ÄZQ) (www.leitlinienmanual.de, accessed 15 September 2012).

AWMF, BÄK, KBV (2010). *NVL Methoden-Report*. Berlin, German Agency for Quality in Medicine (ÄZQ) (http://www.versorgungsleitlinien.de/methodik/pdf/nvl_methode_4.aufl.pdf, accessed 20 August 2012).

ÄZQ (2009). *Programm für Nationale VersorgungsLeitlinien von BÄK, KBV und AWMF. Qualitätsindikatoren – Manual für Autoren*. Berlin, German Agency for Quality in Medicine (ÄZQ) (http://www.aezq.de/mdb/edocs/pdf/schriftenreihe/schriftenreihe36.pdf, accessed 20 August 2012).

ÄZQ (2010). About German disease management guidelines [web site]. Berlin, German Agency for Quality in Medicine (ÄZQ) (http://www.versorgungsleitlinien.de/english, accessed 20 August 2012).

ÄZQ (2011a). Arztbibliothek [German e-health library] [web site]. Berlin, German Agency for Quality in Medicine (ÄZQ) (http://www.arztbibliothek.de/, accessed 20 August 2012).

ÄZQ (2011b). DELBI – German instrument for methodological guideline appraisal [web site]. Berlin, German Agency for Quality in Medicine (ÄZQ) (http://www.leitlinien.de/leitlinienmethodik/leitlinienbewertung/delbi/delbi-english-version, accessed 20 August 2012).

ÄZQ (2012). Übersicht NVL Typ-2-Diabetes [web site]. Berlin, German Agency for Quality in Medicine (ÄZQ) (http://diabetes.versorgungsleitlinien.de/, accessed 20 December 2012).

BÄK Scientific Advisory Board (2010). Richtlinien, Leitlinien, Empfehlungen zur Qualitätssicherung [web site]. Berlin, German Medical Association (BÄK) (http://www.baek.de/page.asp?his=1.120.121, accessed 15 September 2012).

Baker R et al. (2003). Randomised controlled trial of the impact of guidelines, prioritised review criteria and feedback on implementation of recommendations for angina and asthma. *British Journal of General Practice*, 53(489):284–291.

Bakx JC et al. (2003). Relationship between the general practice guidelines for the diagnosis of hypertension and the indication for treatment and practice in the Nijmegen region, the Netherlands, 1983–2001 [in Dutch]. *Nederlands Tijdschrift Voor Geneeskunde*, 147(13):612–615.

Barahona P et al. (2001). Computerising a guideline for the management of diabetes. *International Journal of Medical Informatics*, 64(2–3):275–284.

Baumer EM, Holzer U, Wabro M (2010). Metaleitlinie Version 1.1 – Im Auftrag des Bundesministeriums für Gesundheit [web site]. Vienna, Gesundheit Österreich GmbH (http://www.goeg.at/cxdata/media/download/berichte/metaleitlinie_11.pdf, accessed 21 September 2011).

Bell CM et al. (2000). Methodological issues in the use of guidelines and audit to improve clinical effectiveness in breast cancer in one United Kingdom health region. *European Journal of Surgical Oncology*, 26:130–136. DOI:10.1053/ejso.1999.0755.

Benhamou M et al. (2009). The gap between practice and guidelines in the choice of first-line disease modifying antirheumatic drug in early rheumatoid arthritis: results from the ESPOIR cohort. *Journal of Rheumatology*, 36(5):934–942.

Berndt M, Fischer G (2000). Medizinische Leitlinien: juristische Dimension. *Deutsches Ärzteblatt*, 97(28–19):1942–1944.

Bero LA et al. (2012). The updated clinical guideline development process in Estonia is an efficient method for developing evidence-based guidelines. *Journal of Clinical Epidemiology*, 66(2): 132–139 (http://www.sciencedirect.com/science/article/pii/S089543561200220X, accessed 5 December 2012).

BMG (2009). Bundesqualitätsleitlinie gemäß Bundesgesetz zur Qualität von Gesundheitsleistungen: Disease Management Programm für Diabetes mellitus Typ 2. Vienna, Austrian Federal Ministry of Health (BMG) (http://bmg.gv.at/home/Schwerpunkte/Gesundheitssystem_Qualitaetssicherung/Bundesqualitaetsleitlinien, accessed 20 August 2012).

BMJ (2009). Preferred reporting items for systematic reviews and meta-analyses: the PRISMA statement. *British Medical Journal*, 339:b2535 (http://www.bmj.com/content/339/bmj.b2535.full?view=long&pmid=19622551, accessed 28 January 2013).

Bolter R et al. (2010). Barrieren der Hausarzte gegen Evidenzbasierte Medizin – ein Verstandnisproblem? Eine qualitative Studie mit Hausarzten. *Zeitschrift für Evidenz, Fortbildung und Qualität im Gesundheitswesen*, 104(8–9):661–666.

Boluyt N, Lincke CR, Offringa M (2005). Quality of evidence-based pediatric guidelines. *Pediatrics*, 115(5):1378–1391.

Bouaud J et al. (2001). A before–after study using OncoDoc, a guideline-based decision-support system on breast cancer management: impact upon physician prescribing behaviour. *Studies in Health Technology & Informatics*, 84(Pt 1):420–424.

Brouwers MC et al. (2010a). AGREE II: advancing guideline development, reporting, and evaluation in health care. *Preventive Medicine*, 51(5):421-424.

Brouwers MC et al. (2010b). Development of the AGREE II, part 1: performance, usefulness and areas for improvement. *Canadian Medical Association Journal*, 182(10):1045–1052.

Brouwers MC et al. (2010c). Development of the AGREE II, part 2: assessment of validity of items and tools to support application. *Canadian Medical Association Journal*, 182(10):E472-428.

Bulgarian Ministry of Health (2008). The national program "Medical standards in the Republic of Bulgaria 2008–2010" [in Bulgarian]. Sofia, Ministry of Health of the Republic of Bulgaria (http://bsid-bg.org/upl_doc/NacPrograma_za_MedStandarti.pdf, accessed 20 August 2012).

Bulgarian Ministry of Health (2009). Медицински стандарти [Medical standards] [web site] [in Bulgarian]. Sofia, Ministry of Health of the Republic of Bulgaria (http://www.mh.government.bg/Articles.aspx?lang=bg-BG&pageid=397, accessed 20 August 2012).

Burgers JS, van Everdingen JJ (2004). Evidence-based guideline development in the Netherlands: the EBRO platform. *Nederlands Tijdschrift voor Geneeskunde*, 148(42):2057–2059.

Burgers JS, Cluzeau FA et al. (2003). Characteristics of high-quality guidelines: evaluation of 86 clinical guidelines developed in ten European countries and Canada. *International Journal of Technology Assessment in Health Care*, 19(1):148–157.

Burgers JS, Grol R et al. (2003a). Internationaler Vergleich von 19 Leitlinien-Programmen – eine Übersicht der AGREE Collaboration. *Zeitschrift für ärztliche Fortbildung und Qualitätssicherung*, 97(1):81–88.

Burgers JS, Grol R et al. (2003b). Towards evidence-based clinical practice: an international survey of 18 clinical guideline programs. *International Journal for Quality in Health Care*, 15(1):31–45.

Burgers JS et al. (2002). Inside guidelines: comparative analysis of recommendations and evidence in diabetes guidelines from 13 countries. *Diabetes Care*, 25(11):1933–1939.

Burgers JS et al. (2004). International assessment of the quality of clinical practice guidelines in oncology using the Appraisal of Guidelines and Research and Evaluation Instrument. *Journal of Clinical Oncology*, 22(10):2000–2007.

Burls A (2010). AGREE II – improving the quality of clinical care. *Lancet*, 376(9747):1128–1129.

Busse R et al., eds. (2010). Tackling chronic disease in Europe: strategies, interventions and challenges. Copenhagen, World Health Organization on behalf of the European Observatory on Health Systems and Policies (http://www.euro.who.int/__data/assets/pdf_file/0008/96632/E93736.pdf, accessed 20 August 2012).

Cabana MD et al. (1999). Why don't physicians follow clinical practice guidelines? A framework for improvement. *Journal of the American Medical Association*, 282(15):1458–1465.

Campbell H et al. (1998). Integrated care pathways. *British Medical Journal*, 316(7125):133–137.

Carlsen B, Kjellberg PK (2010). Guidelines: from foe to friend? Comparative interviews with GPs in Norway and Denmark. *BMC Health Services Research*, 10:17.

CBO (2012). Guidelines [web site]. Utrecht, Dutch Institute for Health Care Improvement (CBO) (http://www.cbo.nl/en/Guidelines/, accessed 15 September 2012).

CEBAM (2012). CEBAM Digital library for health [web site]. Leuven, Belgian Centre for Evidence-Based Medicine (http://www.cebam.be/nl/cdlh/Paginas/default.aspx, accessed 20 August 2012).

CeVeAs (2012a). Focus [web site] [in Italian]. Modena, Centro per la Valutazione dell'Efficacia dell'Assistenza Sanitaria (CeVeAs) (http://www.ceveas.it/flex/cm/pages/ServeBLOB.php/L/IT/IDPagina/1, accessed 15 September 2012).

CeVeAs (2012b). Linee guida disponibili on line [Guidelines available online] [web site]. Modena, Centro per la Valutazione dell'Efficacia dell'Assistenza Sanitaria (CeVeAs) (http://www.ceveas.it/flex/cm/pages/ServeBLOB.php/L/IT/IDPagina/65, accessed 15 September 2012).

Chevreul K et al. (2010). France: health system review. *Health Systems in Transition*, 12(6):1–220.

Chevreul K et al. (forthcoming). France. In: Nolte E, Knai C, eds. *Chronic disease management in Europe: an overview of 13 countries*. Cambridge, RAND Europe.

Choudhry NK, Stelfox HT, Detsky AS (2002). Relationships between authors of clinical practice guidelines and the pharmaceutical industry. *Journal of the American Medical Association*, 287(5):612–617.

Clerc I et al. (2011). GPs and clinical practice guidelines: a reexamination. *Medical Care Research and Review*, 68(4):504–518.

CNSMF (2012). Metodologie [Methodology] [web site]. Bucharest, National Centre for Family Medicine (CNSMF) (http://www.ghidurimedicale.ro/index.php?option=com_content&task=view&id=19&Itemid=27&Itemid=48, accessed 15 September 2012).

Cobos A et al (2005). Cost–effectiveness of a clinical decision-support system based on the recommendations of the European Society of Cardiology and other societies for the management of hypercholesterolemia: report of a cluster-randomized trial. *Disease Management & Health Outcomes*, 13(6):421–432.

Conseil Scientifique (2012). Composition CS [web site]. Luxembourg, Conseil Scientifique Domaine de la Santé (http://www.conseil-scientifique.lu/index.php?id=56, accessed 15 September 2012).

Council of Europe (2001). *Recommendation Rec(2001)13 of the Committee of Ministers to member states on developing a methodology for drawing up guidelines on best medical practices.* Strasbourg, Council of Europe (https://wcd.coe.int/wcd/ViewDoc.jsp?id=228755&BackColorInternet=9999CC&BackColorIntranet=FFBB55&BackColorLogged=FFAC75, accessed 20 August 2012).

Davis DA, Taylor-Vaisey A (1997). Translating guidelines into practice. A systematic review of theoretic concepts, practical experience and research evidence in the adoption of clinical practice guidelines. *Canadian Medical Association Journal*, 157(4):408–416.

DDG (2012). Deutsche Diabetes Gesellschaft [web site]. Berlin, Deutsche Diabetes Gesellschaft (http://www.deutsche-diabetes-gesellschaft.de/, accessed 20 August 2012).

De Bleser L et al. (2006). Defining pathways. *Journal of Nursing Management*, 2006, 14(553–563).

Degen RM, Hodgins JL, Bhandari M (2008). The language of evidence based medicine: answers to common questions? *Indian Journal of Orthopaedics*, 42(2):111–117.

Delgado-Noguera M et al. (2009). Quality assessment of clinical practice guidelines for the prevention and treatment of childhood overweight and obesity. *European Journal of Pediatrics*, 168(7):789–799.

De Marco R et al. (2005). Are the asthma guideline goals achieved in daily practice? A population-based study on treatment adequacy and the control of asthma. *International Archives of Allergy and Immunology*, 138(3):225–234.

Department of Health (2001). *National service framework for diabetes.* Richmond, The National Archives (http://www.dh.gov.uk/en/Publicationsandstatistics/Publications/PublicationsPolicyAndGuidance/Browsable/DH_4096591, accessed 15 September 2011).

Department of Health Promotion and Disease Prevention (2010). *A strategy for the prevention and control of noncommunicable disease in Malta.* Valletta, Maltese Ministry for Health, the Elderly and Community Care and Progress

Press Company Ltd. (http://www.google.co.uk/url?sa=t&source=web&cd=1&ved =0CCEQFjAA&url=https%3A%2F%2Fehealth.gov.mt%2Fdownload. aspx%3Fid%3D4793&rct=j&q=Malta%20Non-Communicable%20 Disease%20Plan&ei=-3h4Tu-OMsir8QOms4DpDA&usg=AFQjCN HuICMbMnVo4a0cNpR9gvc03F_kkQ&cad=rja, accessed 20 September 2011).

Devroey D et al. (2004). A review of the treatment guidelines on the management of low levels of high-density lipoprotein cholesterol. *Cardiology*, 102(2):61–66.

DGS (2012). Mais informação, mais saúde [More information, more health] [web site]. Lisbon, Directorate-General for Health (DGS) of the Portuguese Ministry of Health (http://www.dgs.pt/, accessed 15 September 2012).

Dijkstra RF et al. (2006). Patient-centred and professional-directed implementation strategies for diabetes guidelines: a cluster-randomized trial-based cost–effectiveness analysis. *Diabetic Medicine*, 23(2):164–170.

Dousis E et al. (2008). Practice guidelines in Greek operating theatres. *Health Science Journal*, 2(4):226–233 (http://www.hsj.gr/volume2/issue4/6operating226_233.pdf, accessed 15 September 2012).

Duodecim (2011a). *Current care. Criteria for assessing the guideline topic proposal.* Helsinki, Finnish Medical Society Duodecim (http://www.kaypahoito.fi/khhaku/DocumentDownload?id=e2db59c9-1ad0-11df-95c8-7d14d97c9dbd/PRIO-tool.pdf. accessed 31 October 2012).

Duodecim (2011b). *The Finnish Medical Society Duodecim.* Helsinki, Finnish Medical Society Duodecim (http://www.duodecim.fi/kotisivut/docs/f1908623236/esite_engl_web.pdf, accessed 15 September 2012).

Duodecim (2012). Current care guidelines [web site]. Helsinki, Finnish Medical Society Duodecim (http://www.kaypahoito.fi/web/english/home, accessed 15 September 2012).

EHIF (2012). Estonian Health Insurance Fund [web site]. Tallinn, Estonian Health Insurance Fund (http://www.haigekassa.ee/eng/, accessed 15 September 2012).

EndoDiab (2012). EndoDiab [web site]. Ljubljana, DZS & ZES (http://www.endodiab.si/home/, accessed 20 August 2012).

Ernst A, Kinnear M, Hudson S (2005). Quality of prescribing: a study of guideline adherence of medication in patients with diabetes mellitus. *Practical Diabetes International*, 22(8):285–290.

ESF (2012) *Implementation of medical research in clinical practice.* Strasbourg, European Science Foundation (http://www.esf.org/index.php?id=5971, accessed 28 January 2013).

EUnetHTA (2012). EUnetHTA [web site]. Copenhagen, European Network for Health Technology Assessment (http://www.eunethta.eu/, accessed 20 August 2012).

Evensen AE et al. (2010). Trends in publications regarding evidence-practice gaps: a literature review. *Implementation Science*, 5:11.

Federici A et al. (2006). Colorectal cancer screening: recommendations and guideline adherence by physicians from digestive endoscopy centers in the Lazio region, Italy. *Preventive Medicine*, 43(3):183–186.

Field MJ, Lohr KN, eds. (1990). *Clinical practice guidelines: directions for a new program.* Washington, DC, Institute of Medicine and National Academy Press.

Forýtková L, Bourek A, eds. (2006). *Programy kvality a standardy léčebných postupů, Editorství Standardů léčebných postupů. [Programmes of quality and standards of medical procedures].* Prague, Dashofer Verlag.

Forýtková L, Bourek A, eds. (2008). *Standardy léčebných postupů a Kvalita ve zdravotnictví 2008–2011 [Standards of health care and quality in medicine, 2008 to 2011].* Prague, Dashofer Verlag.

FPS (2012). EvidenceBasedNursing [web site] [in French or Dutch]. Brussels, Belgian Federal Public Service Health, Food Chain Safety and Environment (http://www.health.belgium.be/eportal/Healthcare/healthcareprofessions/Nursingpractitioners/EvidenceBasedNursing/index.htm, accessed 20 August 2012).

Francke AL et al. (2008). Factors influencing the implementation of clinical guidelines for health care professionals: a systematic meta-review. *BMC Medical Informatics and Decision Making*, 8:38.

Frijling BD et al. (2002). Multifaceted support to improve clinical decision making in diabetes care: a randomized controlled trial in general practice. *Diabetic Medicine*, 19(10):836–842.

Gaebel W et al. (2005). Schizophrenia practice guidelines: international survey and comparison. *British Journal of Psychiatry*, 187:248–255.

Ganten JU, Raspe HH (2003). Inpatient medical rehabilitation in diabetes mellitus in light of evidence based practice guidelines: an evaluation on the basis of BfA routine data [in German]. *Die Rehabilitation*, 42(2):94–108.

German Federal Law Gazette (1994). Verordnung über das Verfahren zum Risikostrukturausgleich in der gesetzlichen Krankenversicherung (Risikostruktur-Ausgleichsverordnung – RSAV). *Bundesgesetzblatt I*, 3 January 1994: 5 (http://www.buzer.de/gesetz/3311/a46394.htm?m=diabetes#hit, accessed 20 August 2012).

German Federal Law Gazette (2004). Gesundheitsreformgesetz. *Bundesgesetzblatt I*, 179/2004.

G-I-N (2010). Country update – the Netherlands [web site]. Berlin, Guidelines International Network, German Agency for Quality in Medicine (ÄZQ) (http://www.g-i-n.net/newsletter/country-updates/the-netherlands-february-2010, accessed 15 September 2012).

G-I-N (2012). Introduction [web site]. Berlin, Guidelines International Network, German Agency for Quality in Medicine (ÄZQ) (http://www.g-i-n.net/about-g-i-n, accessed 20 August 2012).

Giorgi R et al. (2001). Elaboration and formalization of current scientific knowledge of risks and preventive measures illustrated by colorectal cancer. *Methods of Information in Medicine*, 40(4):323–330.

Giotto Movement (2012). MovimentoGiotto. Giovani Medici di Medicina Generale [Giotto Movement. Young general practitioners] [web site]. Rome, Vasco da Gama (WONCA Europe) (http://dottorgiotto.altervista.org/nuovo2/index.php, accessed 15 September 2012).

Gitt AK et al. (2011). Adherence of hospital-based cardiologists to lipid guidelines in patients at high risk for cardiovascular events (2L registry). *Clinical Research in Cardiology*, 100(4):277–287.

Glaab T et al. (2006a). Guideline conformance for outpatient management of COPD in Germany [in German]. *Deutsche Medizinische Wochenschrift* (1946), 131(21):1203–1208.

Glaab T et al. (2006b). National survey of guideline-compliant COPD management among pneumologists and primary care physicians. *Journal of Chronic Obstructive Pulmonary Disease*, 3(3):141–148.

GÖG (2012). Quality of processes and structures [web site]. Vienna, Gesundheit Österreich GmbH (http://www.goeg.at/en/QP, accessed 20 August 2012).

Graham ID et al. (2000). A comparison of clinical practice guideline appraisal instruments. *International Journal of Technology Assessment in Health Care*, 16(4):1024–1038.

Grilli R et al. (2000). Practice guidelines developed by specialty societies: the need for a critical appraisal. *Lancet*, 355(9198):103–106.

Grimshaw JM, Russell IT (1993). Effect of clinical guidelines on medical practice: a systematic review of rigorous evaluations. *Lancet*, 342(8883):1317–1322.

Grimshaw JM et al. (2004). Effectiveness and efficiency of guideline dissemination and implementation strategies. *Health Technology Assessment*, 8(6):iii–iv, 1–72.

GuíaSalud (2012a). Biblioteca de Guías de Práctica Clínica del Sistema Nacional de Salud [Clinical practice library for the Spanish national health system] [web site]. Zaragoza, GuíaSalud Biblioteca (http://portal.guiasalud.es/web/guest/home, accessed 20 August 2012).

GuíaSalud (2012b). Catálogo de Guías de Práctica Clínica en el Sistema Nacional de Salud (SNS) [Catalogue of clinical practice guidelines in the national health system] [web site]. Zaragoza, GuíaSalud Biblioteca, 2012 (http://portal.guiasalud.es/web/guest/catalogo-gpc, accessed 20 August 2012).

GuíaSalud (2012c). Guías de Práctica Clínica. Metodología para el desarrollo de Guías de Práctica Clínica [Guidelines for clinical practice. Methodology for the development of clinical practice guidelines] [web site]. Zaragoza, GuíaSalud Biblioteca, 2012 (http://portal.guiasalud.es/web/guest/metodologia-gpc, accessed 20 August 2012).

Gupta M (2011). Improved health or improved decision making? The ethical goals of EBM. *Journal of Evaluation in Clinical Practice*, 17(5):957–963.

Guyatt G (1991). Evidence-based medicine. *ACP Journal Club*, 114(Suppl. 2):A16.

Guyatt G et al. (1992). Evidence-based medicine. A new approach to teaching the practice of medicine. *Journal of the American Medical Association*, 268(17):2420–2425.

Harpole LH et al. (2003). Assessment of the scope and quality of clinical practice guidelines in lung cancer. *Chest*, 123(Suppl. 1):7–20.

Harrison MB, van den Hoek J (for the Canadian Guideline Adaptation Study Group) (2010). *CAN-IMPLEMENT: a guideline adaptation and implementation planning resource*. Kingston, ON, Queen's University School of Nursing and Canadian Partnership Against Cancer (http://www.cancerview.ca/idc/groups/public/documents/webcontent/canimp_toolkit.pdf, accessed 20 August 2012).

Hartmann M et al. (2008). Is the guideline, 'Management of early rheumatoid arthritis' being followed in a rheumatism center? [in German]. *Deutsche Medizinische Wochenschrift* (1946), 133:1721–1724.

HAS (2010). Methodology guide: recommandations pour la pratique clinique (RPC) [web site]. Saint-Denis La Plaine, French National Authority for Health (HAS) (http://www.has-sante.fr/portail/jcms/c_431294/recommandations-pour-la-pratique-clinique-rpc, accessed 20 August 2012).

HAS (2011). La HAS retire la recommandation de bonne pratique sur le diabète de type 2. Décision du Conseil d'Etat [web site]. Saint-Denis La Plaine, French National Authority for Health (HAS) (http://www.has-sante.fr/portail/jcms/c_1050193/la-has-retire-la-recommandation-de-bonne-pratique-sur-le-diabete-de-type-2, accessed 20 August 2012).

HAS (2012). Ensemble, améliorons la qualité en santé [web site]. Saint-Denis La Plaine, French National Authority for Health (HAS) (http://www.has-sante.fr/portail/jcms/j_5/home, accessed 20 August 2012).

Hasenbein U, Wallesch C, Räbiger J (2003). Ärztliche Compliance mit Leitlinien. Ein Überblick vor dem Hintergrund der Einführung von Disease-Management-Programmen. *Gesundheitsökonomie & Qualitätsmanagement*, 8(363–375).

Hasnain-Wynia R (2006). Is evidence-based medicine patient-centered and is patient-centered care evidence-based? *Health Services Research*, 41(1):1–8.

Heffner JE (1998). Does evidence-based medicine help the development of clinical practice guidelines? *Chest*, 113(Suppl. 3):172–178.

Hermens RP, Hak E, Hulscher ME (2001). Adherence to guidelines on cervical cancer screening in general practice: programme elements of successful implementation. *British Journal of General Practice*, 51(472):897–903.

Hewitt-Taylor J (2006). Evidence-based practice, clinical guidelines and care protocols. In: Hewitt-Taylor J, ed. *Clinical guidelines and care protocols*. Chichester, John Wiley & Sons: 1–16.

HIQA (2011). *Draft national quality assurance criteria for clinical guidelines*. Cork, Health Information and Quality Authority (http://www.hiqa.ie/publications/draft-national-quality-assurance-criteria-clinical-guidelines, accessed 20 August 2012).

HIQA (2012). Safer better care [web site]. Cork, Health Information and Quality Authority (http://www.hiqa.ie, accessed 15 September 2012).

Hormigo Pozo A et al. (2009). Improved effectiveness in the management of cardiovascular risk among type 2 diabetic patients in primary health care [in Spanish]. *Atencion Primaria*, 41(5):240–245.

IQWiG (2011). *Systematische Leitlinienrecherche und -bewertung sowie Extraktion neuer und relevanter Empfehlungen für das DMP Diabetes mellitus Typ 2. Abschlussbericht V09-04.* Cologne, Institut für Qualität und Wirtschaftlichkeit im Gesundheitswesen (https://www.iqwig.de/download/V09-04_Abschlussbericht_Leitlinienrecherche_und-bewertung_fuer_das_DMP_Diabetes_mellitus_Typ_2.pdf, accessed 28 January 2013).

ISS-SNLG (2002). SNLG method. Methodological handbook – how to produce, disseminate and update clinical practice recommendations [web site]. Rome, National Guidelines System (SNLG) and Italian National Institute of Health (ISS) (http://www.snlg-iss.it/en_SNLG_methodological_handbook, accessed 15 September 2012).

ISS-SNLG (2007). *Indicatori per la valutazione di adesione alla LG. I – Manuale d'uso per le Aziende [Indicators for the evaluation of adherence to the guidelines – Manual for companies].* Rome, National Guidelines System (SNLG) and Italian National Institute of Health (ISS) (http://www.snlg-iss.it/cms/files/indicatori%20di%20qualita_toscana.pdf, accessed 15 September 2012).

ISS-SNLG (2009). National guidelines [web site]. Rome, National Guidelines System (SNLG), Italian National Institute of Health (ISS), and National epidemiology, surveillance and health promotion Centre (CNESPS) (http://www.snlg-iss.it/en_national_guidelines#, accessed 15 September 2012).

ISS-SNLG (2012). Goal [web site]. Rome, National Guidelines System (SNLG) and Italian National Institute of Health (ISS) (http://goal.snlg.it/, accessed 15 September 2012).

Juul L et al. (2009). Adherence to guidelines in people with screen-detected type 2 diabetes, ADDITION, Denmark Exemplified by treatment initiation with an ACE inhibitor or an angiotensin-II receptor antagonist. *Scandinavian Journal of Primary Health Care*, 27(4):223–231.

Kamposioras K et al. (2008). Cancer screening in Greece. Guideline awareness and prescription behavior among Hellenic physicians. *European Journal of Internal Medicine*, 19(6):452–460.

Kamyar M et al. (2008). Adherence to clinical guidelines in the prevention of coronary heart disease in type II diabetes mellitus. *Pharmacy World and Science*, 30(1):120–127.

Karbach U et al. (2011). Physicians' knowledge of and compliance with guidelines: an exploratory study in cardiovascular diseases. *Deutsches Arzteblatt International*, 108(5):61–69.

KCE (2011). A propos du KCE [web site]. Brussels, Centre Fédéral d'Expertise des Soins de Santé (KCE) (https://kce.fgov.be/fr/content/a-propos-du-kce, accessed 20 August 2012).

KNGF (2012). KNGF evidence-based clinical practice guidelines [web site]. Amersfoort, Royal Dutch Society for Physical Therapy (KNGF) (https://www.kngfrichtlijnen.nl/654/KNGF-Guidelines-in-English.htm, accessed 15 September 2012).

Kuchler R et al. (2007). Integrierte Versorgung KHK und Diabetes mellitus [Comprehensive care CVD and diabetes mellitus]. *Herz*, 32(8):607–617.

Kuilboer MM et al. (2006). Computed critiquing integrated into daily clinical practice affects physicians' behavior: a randomized clinical trial with asthma critic. *Methods of Information in Medicine*, 45(4):447–454.

Lagerlov P et al. (2000a). Asthma management in five European countries: doctors' knowledge, attitudes and prescribing behaviour. *European Respiratory Journal*, 15(1):25–29.

Lagerlov P et al. (2000b). Improving doctors' prescribing behaviour through reflection on guidelines and prescription feedback: a randomised controlled study. *Quality in Health Care*, 9(3):159–165.

L'Assurance Maladie (2010). *CAPI. Programme d'evolution des pratiques*. Paris, L'Assurance Maladie (http://www.ameli.fr/fileadmin/user_upload/documents/capi-brochure.pdf, accessed 20 August 2012).

Latvian Health Inspectorate (2008). Regulations of the Health Inspectorate [web site]. Riga, Ministry of Health of the Republic of Latvia (http://www.vi.gov.lv/en/start/_142/regulations-of-the-health-inspectorate, accessed 15 September 2012).

Latvian NHS (2012). About NHS [web site]. Riga, Latvian National Health Service (http://www.vmnvd.gov.lv/en/about-nhs, accessed 15 September 2012).

Legido-Quigley H et al. (2008). *Assuring the quality of health care in the European Union: a case for action*. Geneva, World Health Organization on behalf of the European Observatory on Health Systems and Policies (http://www.euro.who.int/__data/assets/pdf_file/0007/98233/E91397.pdf, accessed 20 August 2012).

Libra (2002). Il progetto Libra [The Libra project] [web site]. Ferrara, Linee guida Italiane BPCO, Rinite, Asma (Libra) (http://www.progettolibra.it/, accessed 15 September 2012).

Lindström J et al. (2010). Take action to prevent diabetes – the IMAGE toolkit for the prevention of type 2 diabetes in Europe. *Hormone & Metabolic Research*, 42(Suppl. 1):37–55.

Lohr KN (1990). Institute of Medicine activities related to the development of practical guidelines. *Journal of Dental Education*, 54(11):699–704.

Lohr KN (1994). Guidelines for clinical practice: applications for primary care. *International Journal for Quality in Health Care*, 6(1):17–25.

Lub R et al. (2006). The impact of new insights and revised practice guidelines on prescribing drugs in the treatment of type 2 diabetes mellitus. *British Journal of Clinical Pharmacology*, 62(6):660–665.

Lugtenberg M, Burgers JS, Westert GP (2009). Effects of evidence-based clinical practice guidelines on quality of care: a systematic review. *Quality & Safety in Health Care*, 18(5):385–392.

Lundborg CS et al. (2000). GPs' knowledge and attitudes regarding treatment of UTI and asthma in Sweden: a randomised controlled educational trial on guideline implementation. *European Journal of Public Health*, 10(4):241–246.

Manchon-Walsh P et al. (2011). Variability in the quality of rectal cancer care in public hospitals in Catalonia (Spain): clinical audit as a basis for action. *European Journal of Surgical Oncology*, 37(4):325–333.

Martens JD et al. (2006). Does a joint development and dissemination of multidisciplinary guidelines improve prescribing behaviour? A pre/post study with concurrent control group and a randomised trial. *BMC Health Services Research*, 2(6):145.

Martens JD et al. (2007). The effect of computer reminders on GPs' prescribing behaviour: a cluster-randomised trial. *International Journal of Medical Informatics*, 76:403–416.

Mayer D (2006). Evidence-based medicine. *Epilepsia*, 47(Suppl. 1):3–5.

McDonald CJ (1996). Medical heuristics: the silent adjudicators of clinical practice. *Annals of Internal Medicine*, 124(1 Pt 1):56–62.

McGlynn EA, Kosecoff J, Brook RH (1990). Format and conduct of consensus development conferences. Multi-nation comparison. *International Journal of Technology Assessment in Health Care*, 6(3):450–469.

McQueen MJ (2001). Overview of evidence-based medicine: challenges for evidence-based laboratory medicine. *Clinical Chemistry*, 47(8):1536–1546.

Meulepas MA et al. (2007). Logistic support service improves processes and outcomes of diabetes care in general practice. *Family Practice*, 24(1):20–25.

Muche-Borowski C, Kopp I (2011). Wie eine Leitlinie entsteht. *Zeitschrift für Herz-, Thorax- und Gefäßchirurgie*, 25(4):217–223.

Nagel H, Baehring T, Scherbaum WA (2006). Implementing disease management programmes for type 2 diabetes in Germany. *Managed Care*, 15(11):50–53.

Nagy E et al. (2008). Do guidelines for the diagnosis and monitoring of diabetes mellitus fulfill the criteria of evidence-based guideline development? *Clinical Chemistry*, 54(11):1872–1882.

National Institute for Strategic Health Research (2011). January 2011. *Hungarian Health System Scan*, 4(1): 1–12 (http://www.eski.hu/new3/hirlevel_en/2011/health_system_scan_2011_1.pdf, accessed 15 September 2012).

Navarro Puerto MA et al. (2008). Analysis of the quality of clinical practice guidelines on established ischemic stroke. *International Journal of Technology Assessment in Health Care*, 24(3):333–341.

NHG (2012). Kenniscentrum [Knowledge centre] [web site]. Utrecht, Dutch College of General Practitioners (NHG) (http://nhg.artsennet.nl/kenniscentrum.htm, accessed 15 September 2012).

NHS Choices (2012). National service frameworks and strategies [web site]. London, National Health Service (http://www.nhs.uk/nhsengland/NSF/pages/Nationalserviceframeworks.aspx, accessed 20 August 2012).

NICE (2009a). *Media statement. Judgement in favour of NICE on judicial review of abatacept for rheumatoid arthritis guidance.* London, National Institure for Clinical Excellence (http://www.nice.org.uk/media/D8D/5C/AbataceptJudicialReviewJudgement.pdf, accessed 20 August 2012).

NICE (2009b). *The guidelines manual 2009* (January 2009). London, National Institute for Health and Clinical Excellence, 2009 (http://www.nice.org.uk/aboutnice/howwework/developingniceclinicalguidelines/clinicalguidelinedevelopmentmethods/GuidelinesManual2009.jsp, accessed 20 August 2012).

NICE (2010). Measuring the use of NICE guidance [web site]. London, National Institute for Health and Clinical Excellence (http://www.nice.org.uk/usingguidance/evaluationandreviewofniceimplementationevidenceernie/evaluation_and_review_of_nice_implementation_evidence_ernie.jsp, accessed 15 September 2012).

NICE (2011a). Diabetes in adults quality standard (QS6). London, National Institute for Health and Clinical Excellence (http://www.nice.org.uk/guidance/qualitystandards/diabetesinadults/diabetesinadultsqualitystandard.jsp, accessed 15 September 2011).

NICE (2011b). NICE implementation uptake report: the management of type 2 diabetes. London, National Institute for Health and Clinical Excellence (http://www.nice.org.uk/media/0BE/AA/UptakeReportCG87Diabetes March2011Publication.pdf, accessed 15 September 2011).

NICE (2011c). *Public health programme – preventing type 2 diabetes: population and community interventions. List of registered stakeholders as of April 2011.* London, National Institute for Health and Clinical Excellence (http://www. nice.org.uk/nicemedia/live/12067/48440/48440.pdf. accessed 15 September 2011).

NICE (2012a). About NICE [web site]. London, National Institute for Health and Clinical Excellence (http://www.nice.org.uk/, accessed 15 September 2012).

NICE (2012b). ERNIE search [web site]. London, National Institute for Health and Clinical Excellence (http://www.nice.org.uk/usingguidance/ measuringtheuseofguidance/searchernie/search_ernie.jsp, accessed 28 January 2013).

NICE (2012c). Shared learning: implementing NICE guidance [web site]. London, National Institute for Health and Clinical Excellence (http://www. nice.org.uk/usingguidance/sharedlearningimplementingniceguidance/shared_ learning_implementing_nice_guidance.jsp, accessed 15 September 2012).

NICE Pathways (2011). Diabetes overview [web site]. London, National Institute for Health and Clinical Excellence (http://pathways.nice.org.uk/ pathways/diabetes, accessed 15 September 2011).

NIKI (2005a). *A guideline developers' handbook.* Bratislava, Interaction in Health, AGIS, University of Amsterdam, Trnava University and Bratislava Health Management School (http://www.quality.healthnet.sk/EBM/ Guidelines_development_handbook Slovak_version_v1 pdf, accessed 15 September 2012).

NIKI (2005b). Project abstract [web site]. Bratislava, National Institute of Quality and Innovation (NIKI) (http://www.niki.healthnet.sk/NIKI_eng/ index.htm, accessed 15 September 2012).

Nolte E, Knai C, McKee M (2008). *Managing chronic diseases. Experience in eight countries.* Copenhagen, World Health Organization on behalf of the European Observatory on Health Systems and Policies (http://www.euro.who. int/__data/assets/pdf_file/0008/98414/E92058.pdf, accessed 15 September 2012).

NRC (2012). Národní referenční centrum [National Reference Centre] [web site]. Prague, National Reference Centre (http://www.nrc.cz/en, accessed 15 September 2012).

Ollenschläger G (2007). Nicht linientreu. Die Entwicklung Nationaler VersorgungsLeitlinien von BÄK, KBV und AWMF schreitet gut voran. *Niedersächsisches Ärzteblatt*, 80(6):48–49.

Pajunen P et al. (2010). Quality indicators for the prevention of type 2 diabetes in Europe – IMAGE. *Hormone & Metabolic Research*, 42(Suppl. 1):56–63.

Paulweber B et al. (2010). A European evidence-based guideline for the prevention of type 2 diabetes. *Hormone & Metabolic Research*, 42(Suppl. 1):3–36.

Perria C et al. (2007). Implementing a guideline for the treatment of type 2 diabetics: results of a cluster-randomized controlled trial (C-RCT). *BMC Health Services Research*, 7:79.

Peters-Klimm F et al. (2008). Guideline adherence for pharmacotherapy of chronic systolic heart failure in general practice: a closer look on evidence-based therapy. *Clinical Research in Cardiology*, 97(4):244–252.

Pont LG et al. (2004). Relationship between guideline treatment and health-related quality of life in asthma. *European Respiratory Journal*, 23(5):718–722.

Ratsep A et al. (2006). Family doctors' knowledge and self-reported care of type 2 diabetes patients in comparison to the clinical practice guideline: cross-sectional study. *BMC Family Practice*, 16(7):36.

Regieraad Kwaliteit van Zorg (2012). *Working on the quality of health care*. The Hague, Dutch Council for the Quality of Health Care (http://www.regieraad.nl/fileadmin/www.regieraad.nl/publiek/048_009_FLYER_02.pdf, accessed 15 September 2012).

RIVM (2012). National Institute for Public Health and the Environment [web site]. Bilthoven, National Institute for Public Health and the Environment (RIVM) of the Ministry of Health, Welfare and Sport of the Netherlands (http://www.rivm.nl/en/, accessed 15 September 2012).

Rosemann T et al. (2007). Case management of arthritis patients in primary care: a cluster-randomized controlled trial. *Arthritis & Rheumatism*, 57(8):1390–1397.

Sackett DL et al. (1996). Evidence-based medicine: what it is and what it isn't. *British Medical Journal* (Clinical Research ed.), 312(7023):71–72.

Sarc I et al. (2011). Adherence to treatment guidelines and long-term survival in hospitalized patients with chronic obstructive pulmonary disease. *Journal of Evaluation in Clinical Practice*, 17(4):737–743.

Schaapveld M et al. (2005). Guideline adherence for early breast cancer before and after introduction of the sentinel node biopsy. *British Journal of Cancer*, 93(5):520–528.

Schafer I et al. (2010). The disease management program for type 2 diabetes in Germany enhances process quality of diabetes care – a follow-up survey of patients' experiences. *BMC Health Services Research*, 10:55.

Schunemann HJ et al. (2009). A vision statement on guideline development for respiratory disease: the example of COPD. *Lancet*, 373(9665):774–779.

Schwarz PE, Lindström J (2011). From evidence to practice – the IMAGE project – new standards in the prevention of type 2 diabetes. *Diabetes Research & Clinical Practice*, 91(2):138–140.

Schwarz PE et al. (2007). The European perspective on diabetes prevention: development and implementation of a European guideline and training standards for diabetes prevention (IMAGE). *Diabetes & Vascular Disease Research*, 4(4):353–357.

Shekelle PG et al. (1999). Clinical guidelines: developing guidelines. *British Medical Journal*, 318(7183):593–596.

SIGN (2012). Published guidelines [web site]. Edinburgh, Scottish Intercollegiate Guidelines Network (http://www.sign.ac.uk/guidelines/published/numlist.html, accessed 2 February 2012).

Sinnema H et al. (2011). Randomised controlled trial of tailored interventions to improve the management of anxiety and depressive disorders in primary care. *Implementation Science*, 6:75.

SIQuAS (2012). The SIQuAS-allele [web site]. Milan, Italian Society for Quality in Health Care (SIQuAS-allele) (http://www.siquas.it/, accessed 15 September 2012).

Slovenian Ministry of Health (2003). *Manual on development of clinical practice guidelines.* Ljubljana, Ministry of Health of the Republic of Slovenia (http://www.mz.gov.si/fileadmin/mz.gov.si/pageuploads/mz_dokumenti/delovna_podrocja/zdravstveno_varstvo/kakovost/prirocniki_in_publikacije/prirocnik_za_smernice_slo.pdf, accessed 20 August 2012).

Smith BJ et al. (2003). Systematic assessment of clinical practice guidelines for the management of chronic obstructive pulmonary disease. *Respiratory Medicine*, 97(1):37–45.

Smith CJP et al. (2008). The impact of the 2004 NICE guideline and 2003 General Medical Services contract on COPD in primary care in the UK. *Quarterly Journal of Medicine*,101(2):145–153.

Smolders M et al. (2009). Adherence to evidence-based guidelines for depression and anxiety disorders is associated with recording of the diagnosis. *General Hospital Psychiatry*, 31(5):460–469.

Smolders M et al. (2010). Which physician and practice characteristics are associated with adherence to evidence-based guidelines for depressive and anxiety disorders? *Medical Care*, 48(3):240–248.

Socialstyrelsen (2011). About the Swedish National Board of Health and Welfare guidelines [web site]. Stockholm, Swedish National Board of Health and Welfare (http://www.socialstyrelsen.se/nationalguidelines/abouttheguidelines, accessed 20 August 2012).

Socialstyrelsen (2012). The National Board of Health and Welfare [web site]. Stockholm, Swedish National Board of Health and Welfare (http://www. socialstyrelsen.se/english, accessed 28 January 2013).

Sondergaard J et al. (2002). Detailed postal feedback about prescribing to asthma patients combined with a guideline statement showed no impact: a randomised controlled trial. *European Journal of Clinical Pharmacology*, 58(2):127–132.

Spencer E, Walshe K (2009). National quality improvement policies and strategies in European healthcare systems. *Quality & Safety in Health Care*, 18(Suppl_1):i22–i27.

Stone MA et al. (2010). Evaluation and comparison of guidelines for the management of people with type 2 diabetes from eight European countries. *Diabetes Research and Clinical Practice*, 87(2):252–260.

Subata E (2009). History, methods and implementation of national treatment guidelines. In: Jasaitis E. *National report (2009 data) to the EMCDDA by the Reitox National Focal Point. Lithuania: new development, trends and in-depth information on selected issues*. Vilnius, The Drug Control Department under the Government of the Republic of Lithuania: 91 (http://www.ntakd.lt/files/ informacine_medzega/1-NKD_medziaga/1-metiniai_pranesimai/Lithuania_ National_report_to_the_EMCDDA_2010.pdf, accessed 15 September 2012).

Tabrizi JS (2009). Quality of delivered care for people with type 2 diabetes: a new patient-centred model. *Journal of Research in Health Sciences*, 9(2):1–9.

The Cochrane Collaboration (2012). Working together to provide the best evidence for health care [web site]. Oxford, The Cochrane Collaboration (http://www.cochrane.org/, accessed 20 August 2012).

THL (2012). National Institute for Health and Welfare [web site]. Helsinki, Finnish National Institute for Health and Welfare (http://www.thl.fi/en_US/web/en/home, accessed 20 August 2012).

Thornhill M et al. (2011). Impact of the NICE guideline recommending cessation of antibiotic prophylaxis for prevention of infective endocarditis: before and after study. *British Medical Journal*, 342:DOI 10.1136/bmj.d2392.

Tinelli C et al. (2003). Evaluation of the efficacy of the Italian guidelines on COPD: a cluster randomized trial. *Monaldi archives for chest disease = Archivio Monaldi per le malattie del torace / Fondazione clinica del lavoro, IRCCS [and] Istituto di clinica tisiologica e malattie apparato respiratorio, Università di Napoli, Secondo ateneo*, 3:199–206 (http://www.mrw.interscience.wiley.com/cochrane/clcentral/articles/141/CN-00471141/frame.html, accessed 20 August 2012).

Toti F et al. (2007). Poor control and management of cardiovascular risk factors among Albanian diabetic adult patients. *Primary Care Diabetes*, 1(2):81–86.

Tsagaraki, V, Markantonis SL, Amfilochiou A (2006). Pharmacotherapeutic management of COPD patients in Greece – adherence to international guidelines. *Journal of Clinical Pharmacy and Therapeutics*, 31(4):369–374.

UGENT, UCL (2012). Nursing scales and guidelines [web site]. Brussels, Ghent University, University College London and Louvain Catholic University (http://www.nursingscales-guidelines.be/FR/index.html, accessed 20 August 2012).

Vale L et al. (2007). Systematic review of economic evaluations and cost analyses of guideline implementation strategies. *European Journal of Health Economics*, 8(2):111–121. Epub 2007/03/10.

Van Bruggen R et al. (2008). Implementation of locally adapted guidelines on type 2 diabetes. *Family Practice*, 25(6):430–437.

Van Steenbergen LN et al. (2009). Improvable quality of diagnostic assessment of colorectal cancer in southern Netherlands. *European Journal of Gastroenterology and Hepatology*, 21(5):570–575.

Varga D et al. (2010). Does guideline-adherent therapy improve the outcome for early-onset breast cancer patients? *Oncology*, 78:189–195.

Vergnenegre A (2003). Clinical practice guidelines: a reader's guide [in French]. *Revue des Maladies Respiratoires*, 20(6 (pt 1)):920–927.

Verlagshaus der Ärzte (2012). EbM-Guidelines. Die Online-Version [web site]. Vienna, Verlagshaus der Ärzte (http://www.ebm-guidelines.at/index.php?&cm s=1&akt=70&sub1=52&sub2=58&sub3=70, accessed 20 August 2012).

Verstappen WH et al. (2003). Effect of a practice-based strategy on test ordering performance of primary care physicians: a randomized trial. *Journal of the American Medical Association*, 289(18):2407–2412.

Vlayen J et al. (2005). A systematic review of appraisal tools for clinical practice guidelines: multiple similarities and one common deficit. *International Journal for Quality in Health Care*, 17(3):235–242.

Voellinger R et al. (2003). Major depressive disorder in the general hospital: adaptation of clinical practice guidelines. *General Hospital Psychiatry*, 25(3):185–193.

Wagner N et al. (2004). The use of guidelines in the primary care management of hypertension and diabetes [in German]. *Sozial- und Praventivmedizin*, 49(4):261–268.

Waldmann A et al. (2007). Description of the medical care of younger patients (< 65 years) with colorectal cancer in Schleswig-Holstein – are diagnostics and therapy compliant with the actual S3-guidelines? [in German]. *Gesundheitswesen*, 69(4):216–223.

Ward JE, Grieco V (1996). Why we need guidelines for guidelines: a study of the quality of clinical practice guidelines in Australia. *Medical Journal of Australia*, 165(10):574–576.

Watine JC, Bunting PS (2008). Mass colorectal cancer screening: methodological quality of practice guidelines is not related to their content validity. *Clinical Biochemistry*, 41(7–8):459–466.

Wennberg J, Gittelsohn J (1973). Small area variations in health care delivery. *Science (New York)*, 182(4117):1102–1108.

Wennekes L et al. (2008). Possibilities for transborder cooperation in breast cancer care in Europe: a comparative analysis regarding the content, quality and evidence use of breast cancer guidelines. *Breast*, 17(5):464–471.

Wiener-Ogilvie S et al. (2007). Do practices comply with key recommendations of the British Asthma Guideline? If not, why not? *Primary Care Respiratory Journal*, 16(6):369–377. Epub 6.

Winnefeld M, Bruggemann S (2008). Practice guideline for breast cancer rehabilitation from the perspective of the rehabilitation centres: findings of a user survey on acceptance and practicability of the pilot version [in German]. *Die Rehabilitation*, 47(6):334–342.

Witt K et al. (2004). Academic detailing has no effect on prescribing of asthma medication in Danish general practice: a 3-year randomized controlled trial with 12-monthly follow-ups. *Family Practice*, 21(3):248–253.

Wockel A et al. (2010). Effects of guideline adherence in primary breast cancer. A 5-year multi-center cohort study of 3976 patients. *Breast*, 19(2):120–127.

Woolf SH et al. (1999). Clinical guidelines: potential benefits, limitations, and harms of clinical guidelines. *British Medical Journal*, 318(7182):527–530.

Zink A, Huscher D, Schneider M (2010). How closely does rheumatology treatment follow the guidelines? Ambition and reality [in German]. *Zeitschrift fur Rheumatologie*, 69(4):318–326.

EU Member States' use of guidelines

Country	Definition and regulatory basis	Types and levels	Actors involved	Development process
Austria	Clinical guidelines are developed by national societies of medical specialists and Federal Quality Guidelines are broader recommendations on health service delivery and organization, which incorporate clinical guidelines. The Physicians' Act – a law which distinguishes federal quality directives – is legally binding, and Federal quality guidelines are simply recommendations (not legally blinding).	Clinical guidelines exist for several diseases, in particular for chronic conditions. Most of the clinical guidelines are developed by national societies of medical specialists. Federal quality guidelines have influence at country level.	Clinical guidelines can be developed by national or international societies of medical specialists. Federal quality guidelines are developed by the BIQG, a section of the GmbH. The topic for these guidelines can be suggested by any organization. All relevant stakeholders are involved in their development, including patient representatives.	Guidelines are federally regulated but other (non-official) projects also exist for developing them. Guidance exists for the development and implementation of federal quality guidelines ("meta-guideline"); it is based on international methodology including the AGREE instrument. For the development of clinical guidelines the following issues must be considered: evidence-based medicine, national priorities, health service integration, professional relevance, patient-centredness, health promotion, transparency.

Quality control	Enforcement	Implementation	Evaluation
federal quality guidelines undergo quality control by a pool of experts that also assess financial issues and feasibility. In addition, there is an external review by means of a consensus process, involving the informed public. For clinical guidelines developed by medical associations or expert groups, there is no quality monitoring.	The use of guidelines is not mandatory. As sound and effective tools in patient care, they should serve as a basis for decision-making.	Implementation of federal quality guidelines is driven by the "meta-guideline". So far only one of those guidelines has been implemented (type 2 diabetes mellitus).	According to the "meta-guideline", federal quality guidelines should be evaluated by the respective organization in charge of launching the development of such guidelines. Evaluation should be carried out nationally. Funding for evaluation must be provided by the initiators of the respective guidelines.

Country	Definition and regulatory basis	Types and levels	Actors involved	Development process
Belgium	Some clinical guidelines are adapted from international clinical guidelines (type 2 diabetes mellitus, coronary heart disease, COPD), others are developed nationally, and in some cases (i.e. for arthritis) there is no central coordination of guideline development. However, the country is currently trying to achieve a better coordination of clinical guidelines development by giving legal basis to the EBMPracticeNet (a voluntary platform of national evidence-based medicine organizations that aim to stimulate cooperation and coordination between the different actors).	Clinical guidelines exist for prevention and treatment of several diseases, including chronic conditions. Clinical guidelines can operate at local, regional or national levels.	Several entities – centralized or not – are involved in clinical guidelines development and dissemination: universities, hospitals professional associations, scientific associations (involving practitioners and patients), colleges of medicine, governmental entities. Several structures contribute to the dissemination of clinical guidelines: the colleges of physicians, the KCE, the CEBAM, the BAPCOC, the EBMPracticeNet and the Federal Council for the Quality of Nursing. The composition of the GDG varies across clinical guidelines and organizations. Usually the main participants are clinicians, content experts, and systematic review experts. In governmental settings policy-makers and health economists can also be included. In certain (very specific) guidelines, patient representatives are also being included.	Clinical guidelines development can be initiated by both governmental and other organizations. Clinical guidelines can be funded by the government, or by different organizations. For clinical guidelines funded by national and regional authorities, the topics are sometimes chosen by these authorities. During the past decade the development of clinical guidelines has become more rigorous and evidence-based. However, the involved actors and the methodology used to develop clinical guidelines vary across organizations. Also the approach for retrieving and assessing the evidence varies; it is generally performed by researchers or health care professionals with relevant skills acquired through specific training or education. CEBAM provides open training in evidence-based medicine.

Quality control	Enforcement	Implementation	Evaluation
The validation of clinical guidelines is not mandatory; and there is no standard procedure. CEBAM can be asked to validate clinical guidelines with the AGREE instrument in combination with a limited analysis of the content. The validation procedure results in a decision regarding whether to recommend the clinical guidelines. Sometimes this step is a prerequisite for funding by the government. All guidelines in the field of nursing must be evaluated with the AGREE criteria. Clinical guidelines that have been adapted from other countries are usually tested for applicability in the Belgian context according to the ADAPTE Procedure which is used by various organizations.	The use of guidelines is not mandatory, except in the nursing care setting at hospital level. However, whether certain drugs, therapeutic measures or diagnostic interventions are suitable for individual patients can be established by consulting the instructions provided in the guidelines.	Clinical guidelines dissemination and implementation are not standardized. Developers are in charge of publishing clinical guidelines. The Belgian scientific associations and colleges of physicians disseminate their clinical guidelines through professional papers and medical local press. The CEBAM web site is also used to publish clinical guidelines. A new tool that is to be introduced is the EBMeDS system that brings evidence into practice by means of context-sensitive guidance at the point of care through the electronic patient record.	No formal evaluations are in place with the exception of selected specific topics (i.e. antibiotics). A new system for evaluation of hospital nursing clinical guidelines is being developed. Some colleges of physicians define criteria for evaluation of clinical guidelines and assess them. However, this is not carried out systematically.

Country	Definition and regulatory basis	Types and levels	Actors involved	Development process
Bulgaria	The existing recommendations are: clinical pathways (for treatment of acute episodes of chronic conditions or chronic patients' rehabilitation); NMS (mostly related to conditions to protect practising medical professionals but some also have elements similar to clinical guidelines, such as an algorithm which general practitioners are obliged to follow while managing diabetes). There is a legal basis for the development and implementation of centrally developed guidance.	Clinical guidelines – as defined in this report – are limited and do not encompass all chronic conditions. All legally regulated guidelines are developed centrally. Clinical guidelines on chronic diseases refer to separate episodes of illness and do not embrace the overall management of conditions.	Scientific medical associations and academic societies can be involved in clinical guideline development. The National Health Insurance Fund is responsible for the development of clinical pathways, while Ministry of Health experts develop NMS and methodological guidelines.	Development of clinical guidelines, algorithms and protocols are based on international Bulgarian publications in recognized journals. All guidelines are developed by means of consensus processes supported by current literature. Clinical pathways and NMS are periodically updated. Updates are often initiated by medical professionals, but the Ministry of Health and the National Health Insurance Fund bear responsibility for guideline quality.

Quality control	Enforcement	Implementation	Evaluation
There is no regulated process of clinical guidelines validation.	Clinical guidelines are not mandatory, but NMS are. Clinical pathways are mandatory for hospitals or general practitioners contracted by the National Health Insurance Fund (in order to receive payment).	Clinical guidelines implementation depends on the provider. NMS implementation is controlled by the regional structures of the Ministry of Health.	No formal evaluations are in place. National Health Insurance Fund controls provider compliance with contractual agreements.

Country	Definition and regulatory basis	Types and levels	Actors involved	Development process
Cyprus	Clinical guidelines exist but they are poorly implemented. No other tools are in place to assist professionals in the decision-making process. There is no legal framework or official basis for clinical guidelines development and implementation.	Clinical guidelines sporadically exist.	The Ministry of Health is in charge of developing and implementing clinical guidelines. A parallel role has also been taken on by the National Health Insurance Organization that is responsible for the new NHIS. The NHIS developed committees to deal with relevant clinical guidelines and several clinical guidelines are being developed.	The development of clinical guidelines is not based on evidence-based methodology.
Czech Republic	Since 2009 the NRC is in charge of developing methodologies and implementing NSHS and NHSIS development standards. It is part of the Ministry of Health.	Clinical guidelines exist (and are periodically updated) on coronary heart disease, diabetes, asthma, COPD, and cancer. Over 250 clinical guidelines exist on other conditions.	The process of clinical guidelines development is centralized since the NRC was put in charge of their development. However, there is also a decentralized branch, DASHOFER publishing house, funded by external resources and coordinated by the Center for Healthcare Quality.	Clinical guidelines development is funded by the Ministry of Health and also by external resources. The NRC and DASHOFER collaborate on clinical guidelines development. However, no guidance exists for the development of clinical guidelines.

Quality control	Enforcement	Implementation	Evaluation
There is no regulated process of clinical guidelines validation. The new NHIS includes a proposal to improve the whole process of developing, implementing and evaluating clinical guidelines.	Clinical guidelines are not mandatory and there are no financial incentives for their implementation and use. Based on the new NHIS, financial incentives will be introduced to maximize implementation and use of clinical guidelines. The new NHIS also includes clinical guidelines promotion through IT applications (an electronic disease management system which will be able to document, guide and support the physicians' decision-making process for specific chronic diseases).	Clinical guidelines are poorly implemented.	No regulated evaluation control system is in place.
The AGREE instrument is used for clinical guidelines quality control. For the main standards the quality control is performed by professional medical associations.	The implementation and use of clinical guidelines is not mandatory.	Clinical guidelines are available on several web sites and they are promoted through IT applications.	No regulated evaluation control system is in place. Assessment of adherence to clinical guidelines is carried out on a self-organizing basis.

Country	Definition and regulatory basis	Types and levels	Actors involved	Development process
Denmark	Guidelines and other tools are available to assist professionals with the decision-making process.	Clinical guidelines exist for a range of conditions with an increased emphasis on those for preventing and treating chronic diseases.	Clinical guidelines are developed both centrally and at a decentralized level. The National Board of Health and the Institute for Rational Pharmacotherapy provide guidance at central level. Regional and municipal authorities, professional organizations, nursing associations or medical societies also develop clinical guidelines. The DSAM is involved in the production of central clinical guidelines but also produces its own guidelines.	Clinical guidelines development is not coordinated by any individual institution. Guidance for clinical guidelines development and implementation does not exist.

Quality control	Enforcement	Implementation	Evaluation
There is no regulated process of clinical guidelines validation.	The use of clinical guidelines is not mandatory.	Clinical guidelines implementation is not centrally regulated.	There is no formal evaluation.
The AGREE instrument is often used to assess clinical guidelines quality when guidelines are used for HTA production.		IT applications and Disease Management Programmes are available to support professionals.	However, clinical guidelines use is evaluated within accreditation programmes for publicly funded hospitals.
		However, no guideline database is available.	

Country	Definition and regulatory basis	Types and levels	Actors involved	Development process
Estonia	The EHIF has been coordinating development methodologies since 2003. However, only few clinical guidelines are formally acknowledged by the Fund. Tools other than clinical guidelines are also available to assist professionals, such as white papers for home, school or family nurses.	Clinical guidelines exist for the management of chronic diseases as well as for other conditions. Some clinical guidelines are ex-novo developed while others are translated from foreign guidelines. However, there is no coordination and in some cases several sets of guidelines exist for one condition.	According to an agreement of the EHIF, a number of public institutions in the health system have certain mandates to facilitate or/ and develop clinical guidelines. These are: EHIF, Ministry of Social Affairs, National Institute for Health Development, Estonian e-Health Foundation, providers of health care services, various medical associations, etc.	Clinical guideline development has been coordinated by the EHIF since 2003. Most of the existing clinical guidelines were developed by professional associations and many of those were commissioned by the EHIF. The Ministry of Social Affairs and the National Institute for Health Development have recently commissioned a limited amount of guidelines. Guidance for the development of clinical guidelines has been available since 2003 and a new handbook on clinical guideline methodology was launched in 2011 (Bero et al., 2012). The use of evidence-based methodology is increasing.

Quality control	Enforcement	Implementation	Evaluation
The methodological handbook on clinical guidelines development provides tools for their quality assessment. However, it is unclear which instrument is used.	The use of clinical guidelines is not mandatory. However, the importance of following clinical guidelines is highlighted in the contracts between providers (at both primary care and hospital levels) and the EHIF.	The implementation of clinical guidelines is not methodologically supported but financial incentives are in place. The bonus payment system for quality for general practitioners includes indicators on management of chronic conditions and preventive care. These indicators were developed based on good clinical practice and clinical guidelines. No IT applications exist to support guideline implementation.	The use of clinical guidelines is monitored during clinical audit and by the "trustee doctors" system in place within the EHIF system.

Country	Definition and regulatory basis	Types and levels	Actors involved	Development process
Finland	Clinical guidelines are produced centrally by the Duodecim. While they have no direct legal position, the government supports both their development and implementation. The Käypä hoito Unit of Duodecim (Current Care) drafts nationwide care guidelines to improve quality of care and reduce variations in care practices.	Clinical guidelines exist for the management of chronic diseases (diabetes, asthma, rheumatic disease, cancer), as well as for other conditions. There are national clinical guidelines on over 100 conditions. Most clinical guidelines focus on prevention, and all on treatment.	The Duodecim steers clinical guideline development. Development of clinical guidelines involves the following actors: Current Care Board (led by 15 members representing a range of interest groups plus the Duodecim's management), Current Care working groups (including about 700 voluntary health workers from a range of fields, information specialists and technical editors). Medical specialist societies cooperate with the Duodecim for clinical guidelines development.	Clinical guidelines are mainly funded by the Finnish Government (via the THL). Duodecim produced (and maintains) an in-house manual on clinical guidelines development. This manual is based mainly on AGREE methods and includes the use of GRADE to ensure grading is evidence based. The Current Care Board selects the topics for clinical guidelines based on suggestions from specialist societies. A set of criteria ("PRIO-tool") is used to assess the guideline proposal and to set priorities. A systematic review of the literature is conducted by experienced professional information specialists. Current Care editors then produce the evidence-based Clinical guidelines.

Quality control	Enforcement	Implementation	Evaluation
Clinical guidelines go through a process of quality control before they are published. A draft is assessed by specific interest groups according to the AGREE criteria and revised according to the comments received. Duodecim is in charge of publishing and updating the final version.	The use of clinical guidelines is not mandatory and there are no financial incentives encouraging their use. Guidelines are designed to support physicians in their clinical practice.	Guidelines are widely used in primary care because of ease of access to them. Their use is promoted through IT applications. They are integrated with the EBMeDS system, allowing them to be opened from within the electronic patient record. In addition, summaries, patient versions, PowerPoint slide series and online courses (selectively) are developed.	Since 2011, the THL is responsible for supervising the development, quality and use of clinical guidelines.

Country	Definition and regulatory basis	Types and levels	Actors involved	Development process
France	The HAS is an independent scientific public authority which develops, disseminates and evaluates the implementation of clinical guidelines within the French health care system. The institution of clinical guidelines is established by law as part of the outputs of the HAS.	Clinical guidelines exist for chronic diseases as well as for other conditions. There are three levels of clinical guidelines development: centrally, undertaken by the HAS; regionally, by regional authorities for some conditions; and by individual providers in certain cases.	As defined by HAS, the GDG consists of 15–20 specialists from different disciplines related to the topic, representatives of the patients and/or health system users.	The HAS publishes its methodology for developing clinical guidelines on its web site. The clinical guidelines are required to be evidence based, supported by a literature review. Clinical guidelines drafts are reviewed by a group of 30–50 people (similar composition to the GDG). The drafts are revised according to the provided feedback. The HAS aims for maximum transparency and objectivity by making both the development and the review groups as independent as possible, both editorially and in terms of conflict of interest.

Quality control	Enforcement	Implementation	Evaluation
The Guidelines Commission and the *College de la HAS* have to validate the recommendations before the guidelines are published on the agency web site. An evidence grading system based on study design is used in the guidelines to underpin the evidence base of each recommendation.	The use of clinical guidelines is not mandatory (an initial phase of financial penalties for non-compliance was soon abandoned). General Practitioners are required to follow Professional Practice Assessments, during which they are made aware of clinical guidelines and are requested to compare their practice to them.	Clinical guidelines are disseminated via the HAS web site, scientific publications, and relevant congresses.	Given that guidelines are not mandatory, no official mechanism for evaluation is in place yet. A recent study shows that awareness among practitioners is not particularly high and more active implementation would be necessary to achieve a higher rate of guideline application.

Country	Definition and regulatory basis	Types and levels	Actors involved	Development process
Germany	The AWMF (the umbrella organization of 158 medical societies) has coordinated clinical guidelines development on behalf of the medical associations since 1995. A separate type of guidelines – those of the NVL programme – is coordinated by the AWMF, the BÄK and the KBV via their joint institute, the ÄZQ. These institutions agreed to national standards for clinical guidelines production and implementation based on Council of Europe Recommendation Rec (2001)13.[d]	Clinical guidelines exist for chronic diseases (both for prevention and treatment) as well as for a multitude of other conditions (679 clinical guidelines were available in the AWMF database in June 2011). Chronic diseases in particular have been the target of Disease Management Programmes, implemented nationwide by the statutory health insurance funds in recent years.	The clinical guideline development is both centrally performed and decentralized. The centralized guidelines are those of the NVL, of the BÄK, KBV and AWMF, BÄEK Scientific Advisory Board, Therapy Guidelines of the BÄEK Drug Commission. Decentralized clinical guidelines are developed by the scientific medical societies coordinated by AWMF.	The NVL programme has its own guidance manual. The AWMF and the ÄZQ have a detailed handbook for decentralized guideline production. The utilization of evidence-based guidelines is also firmly rooted in the Social Security Statute V, which delineates the code of conduct for the statutory health insurance.

[d] Council of Europe, 2001.

Quality control	Enforcement	Implementation	Evaluation
Clinical guidelines coordinated by the ÄZQ or AWMF undergo quality assessment before being implemented. The DELBI checklist is used for this purpose; it is based on the AGREE instrument and adapted for the specific setting within the German health care system. The appraisal is performed by methodologists who were not part of the guideline production process. The AWMF categorizes guidelines based on their methodological background using the "S-classification" (S1: lowest level, drawing on expert opinion; S3: highest level, clinical guidelines based on evidence and consensus process). The IQWiG has been mandated to systematically research and evaluate current clinical guidelines in order to pinpoint the necessity for updating the regulation underpinning Disease Management Programmes.	The use of clinical guidelines is not mandatory. However, whether or not treatment was carried out according to official clinical guidelines can be used as an argument during malpractice cases. Financial incentives to implement guidelines are used as part of Disease Management Programme contracts between social insurance and health care providers.	Tools to support implementation are: quality indicator programmes (e.g. the Program for Cross-Sectoral Quality Assurance of the Joint Committee at the AQUA Institute), IT applications in hospitals combined with clinical pathways based on clinical guidelines (still in the early stages). Guidelines are also collected by the German e-Health library.	There is no national agenda on evaluating the implementation and use of clinical guidelines. The National Academy of Family Physicians evaluates clinical guidelines within its scope. Implementation and utilization of clinical guidelines are evaluated within the setting of Disease Management Programme contracts and of guideline-based quality indicator programmes.

Country	Definition and regulatory basis	Types and levels	Actors involved	Development process
Greece	There is no official basis for the development or implementation of clinical guidelines.	Clinical guidelines are still in their infancy in Greece. Recommendations by specialist medical societies exist for diabetes, coronary heart disease, asthma, COPD and rheumatoid arthritis.	Professionals depend very much on their individual efforts to gather the appropriate evidence in order to make informed decisions.	Currently, no development process for clinical guidelines exists. A debate is currently under way to decide who is going to be in charge of developing clinical guidelines.
Hungary	Clinical guidelines development and implementation are not clearly regulated. In 2011, two organizations were designed to coordinate clinical guidelines centrally: the NABHC and the GYEMSZI.	Clinical guidelines exist for preventing chronic diseases as well as for other conditions. The NABHC designed the production of protocols; these can then be used by individual providers as a basis for producing clinical guidelines. Protocols include an introduction about the disease, prevalence/incidence data, data on prevention, diagnosis, symptoms, principles of treatment, rehabilitation, etc.	The Hungarian clinical guidelines system has both centralized and decentralized components: the NABHC provides treatment recommendations or treatment protocols and then providers (hospitals) are responsible for formulating actual clinical guidelines for use in their own establishments.	Until 2011, clinical guidelines development was not methodologically regulated based on central directions. Since March 2011, the NABHC supervises the development and utilization of guidelines according to specialty and determines the validity period of the guidelines. The GYEMSZI is developing a methodological guide to enhance and unify protocols and clinical guidelines.

Quality control	Enforcement	Implementation	Evaluation
here is no uniform process or quality control. he AGREE instrument s available but it is not eported as a tool in the nal edition of the clinical uidelines. here are a few examples f quality control: clinical uidelines for diabetes were alidated through the ADA nd the SIGN evaluation ystems; for clinical uidelines on coronary heart isease, the ESCARDIO valuation system was used; nd for the asthma/COPD linical guidelines the IPCRG valuation system was used.	The use of clinical guidelines is not mandatory and there are no financial incentives related to their use.	Individual clinical guideline initiatives are promoted by web sites, congresses and scientific societies. Generally, IT applications are not used to promote their implementation. Clinical guidelines developed in other countries (in English) are available on local medical societies' web sites.	There is no formal evaluation of the implementation of or adherence to clinical guidelines.
ince March 2011 quality ontrol of protocols s carried out by the YEMSZI using the AGREE strument.	Clinical guidelines formulated by individual providers (hospitals) are mandatory within the establishment in question.	Implementation of clinical guidelines is not clearly regulated or supported, but is the responsibility of individual providers.	There is no formal evaluation of the implementation of or adherence to clinical guidelines. However, there is currently a partnership between the NABHC and the GYEMSZI to set up an evaluation processes in the health sector.

Country	Definition and regulatory basis	Types and levels	Actors involved	Development process
Ireland	Clinical guidelines development and implementation are not clearly regulated. The NCEC has been set up by the Department of Health to formulate a common approach for clinical guidelines development and an approach for national audit.	Only a few clinical guidelines have been nationally developed in Ireland: e.g. for symptomatic breast care. International guidance is mostly used.	Currently the HSE is rolling out 30 specific clinical care programmes at national level, and programmes exist for diabetes, stroke, acute medicine, elective surgery, etc. Those programmes will also be in charge of providing sets of clinical guidelines.	No clear methodology for clinical guidelines development is currently being used. The NCEC is in the process of approving a modified AGREE II tool for clinical guidelines development (with emphasis on common and chronic conditions).
Italy	The development of clinical guidelines and their implementation are regulated by the Ministry of Health through the SNLG, which is part of the ISS (branch of the Ministry of Health). The SNLG collaborates with the Italian Cochrane Centre and with two regional health services. The SNLG is in charge of updating and developing clinical guidelines.	Clinical practice guidelines exist for several chronic conditions, such as diabetes, coronary heart disease, COPD, asthma, arthritis, mental health, dementia, etc. Several clinical guidelines also exist on acute conditions, emergencies, elderly care and many other conditions. National clinical guidelines are regulated by the SNLG and local clinical guidelines are produced by Regional Agencies.	Clinical guidelines in Italy are developed centrally by the SNLG in collaboration with universities, scientific associations, professional associations and Regional Agencies and Departments of Health. National clinical guidelines are also developed by Specialty Societies and Scientific Multi-specialty committees by adapting international clinical guidelines to the local context (i.e. clinical guidelines on stroke, the Italian guidelines for COPD, rhinitis and asthma). Local clinical guidelines are also developed by Regional Agencies.	Clinical guidelines are developed on the basis of a practical guide designed by the SNLG according to the AGREE standards and they are evidence-based. The guide defines the methodology in detail, including the methodology to perform systematic review, to grade the evidence, to monitor indicators, economical and ethical issues related to the clinical guidelines, strategies to implement clinical guidelines and evaluate them.

Quality control	Enforcement	Implementation	Evaluation
Currently, there is no process for quality control. The new tool that is being developed (see column "Development process") contains issues related to quality control.	Clinical guidelines are not mandatory. However, doctors are required to sign up to a college-managed assurance scheme, with resultant heightened awareness of best practice, standardization and clinical guideline adoption.	Implementation of clinical guidelines is currently not clearly regulated. However, private health care providers are required to be accredited with an international accreditation body for payments to be forthcoming.	There is no formal evaluation of the implementation of or adherence to clinical guidelines.
Clinical guidelines quality control has been required by law since 1992 and it is performed using the AGREE instrument. Quality control is assured by the same body and agencies that developed and implemented the guidelines (SNLG or CeVeAs), but there is also a dedicated agency responsible for quality control, the AGENAS. The ISQuA is also partly responsible for clinical guidelines quality control, along with the Italian representative of the ESQH.	The use of clinical guidelines is not mandatory in Italy and there are no direct financial incentives to implement their use. Instead, some specific directives exist, called "Protocols", the use of which is mandatory; these may be designed by local health institutes (e.g. hospitals) or by regional health institutions, in which case they are mandatory for every medical institute in the respective region.	National and regional health institutions finance and support clinical guidelines implementation. Organizations involved in the implementation of clinical guidelines are the CeVeAs and the National Association of Italian General Practitioner Trainees and Young General Practitioners. The clinical guidelines are publicly available online on several web sites. Their implementation and use are also promoted through a special platform called GOAL developed by the ISS.	Evaluation of adherence to clinical guidelines is required by law and the AGENAS is in charge of it.

Country	Definition and regulatory basis	Types and levels	Actors involved	Development process
Latvia	An official legal basis for clinical guidelines development and implementation was adopted in 2010. It aims to improve clinical guidelines quality: it prescribes the procedures for development, evaluation, registration and implementation of guidelines. The CHE (a governmental institution belonging to the Ministry of Health) is in charge of applying the regulation.	Clinical guidelines for the management of chronic conditions exist (i.e. for diabetes mellitus types 1 and 2, for COPD in primary care, for the treatment of autoimmune inflammatory arthritis, for early detection of malignant tumours, etc.).	The 2010 regulation names the associations that are allowed to develop guidelines. These are professional medical organizations (e.g., endocrinologists, cardiologists, pulmonologists, etc.), medical treatment institutions and institutions of higher education that have academic study programmes in medicine.	The development per se is decentralized. A proposal for clinical guidelines development must be submitted to the CHE by the developer association, as well as the draft of the clinical guidelines. No detailed directives exist for clinical guidelines development. According to the 2010 law, clinical guidelines should be evidence-based.
Lithuania	In 2008 a legal basis for clinical guidelines development and implementation was introduced. It provides the basic requirements for diagnostics and treatment guidelines development and implementation. It is also defined that in the absence of clinical guidelines approved by the Ministry of Health the health institutions have to prepare their own protocols to guarantee the quality of health service provision.	Clinical guidelines exist for specific diseases (including diabetes, coronary heart disease, certain cancers, asthma, arthritis, etc.) and they are usually defined as "diagnostics and treatment methodologies". When no national or local guidelines on specific conditions are available, it is recommended to follow WHO guidelines or the recommendations of international physicians' associations.	Clinical guidelines are developed by individual associations, such as universities, research organizations, physicians' professional associations and/ or Ministry of Health working groups. According to the new law, clinical guidelines development should involve close coordination with the Medical Faculties, National Health Insurance Fund, State Pharmaceutical Control Service and Mandatory Health Insurance Service.	The 2008 law defines methodological guidance for clinical guidelines development, including naming the possible initiators, evidence grading, the process of approval by the Ministry of Health, and of dissemination and implementation. The regulation defines the structure of clinical guidelines and that they have to be evidence-based and state the level of evidence on which they are based.

Quality control	Enforcement	Implementation	Evaluation
he CHE is responsible for ssessing the quality of the linical guidelines. he process should involve ie Board of Leading pecialists and the Health ector Council. lowever, no proper istrument is in use for ssessing their quality.	Clinical guidelines are not clearly mandatory. According to the new law, medical institutions should implement clinical guidelines in compliance with their own financial situation. Moreover, the 2009 Medical Treatment Law prescribes that medical treatment should be performed in conformity with clinical guidelines or methodological recommendations.	When the guidelines are approved, they are registered by the CHE and published on the CHE's web site. Their use is generally promoted through professional associations. The planned development of e-Health is expected to improve the availability of clinical guidelines.	There is no proper mechanism for the evaluation of the clinical guidelines, adherence and impact.
draft of the clinical uidelines has to be eviewed by two identified ational universities and ubsequently by specific gencies of the Ministry of lealth. he instrument used for the uality control is not defined.	The use of guidelines approved by the Ministry of Health is mandatory since 2008. The use of clinical guidelines that are not approved but are published in official sources is recommended.	The implementation of clinical guidelines is regulated by the 2008 law, but no details are available.	Evaluation should be performed according to the 2008 law, but no details are available.

Country	Definition and regulatory basis	Types and levels	Actors involved	Development process
Luxembourg	The Conseil Scientifique has a key role in terms of clinical guidelines; it consists of members of the Ministry of Health, the medical examination services department of the social insurance system and different representatives of the associations of physicians and dentists. Besides the Conseil Scientifique, no "official" basis for clinical guideline development and implementation exists in Luxembourg.	Clinical guidelines exist only for a few conditions, for example for cardiovascular and cerebral diseases.	The Conseil Scientifique consists of members of the Ministry of Health, the medical examination services department of the social insurance system and different representatives of the associations of physicians and dentists.	The development of clinical guidelines is centralized (Conseil Scientifique and the Ministry of Health). Specialist groups submit proposals to put specific conditions or treatments on the agenda for guideline development, but this process is neither centralized nor coordinated. No guidance is available to support clinical guidelines development.

Quality control	Enforcement	Implementation	Evaluation
Currently, there is no process for quality control.	The use of clinical guidelines is not mandatory.	The web site of the Conseil Scientifique functions as an information platform and supports professionals and patients in their decision-making processes.	There is no proper mechanism for the evaluation of the adherence to and impact of clinical guidelines.

Country	Definition and regulatory basis	Types and levels	Actors involved	Development process
Malta	There is no official basis for the development or implementation of clinical guidelines. In 2010 the government published the first national Strategy for the Prevention and Control of Noncommunicable Disease.[c] It identified the development and implementation of national evidence-based guidelines on the primary and secondary prevention of NCDs as a priority for action.	Clinical guidelines exist but they focus on acute conditions or exacerbations of chronic diseases. None exist that focus on the prevention or long-term management of chronic diseases. Clinical guidelines in primary care have been developed only recently (just six of them). Medicine protocols used for entitlement purposes within the Government Health Services are developed and implemented nationally by the Medicines Entitlement Unit and some of these cover medicines used in the treatment of chronic diseases.	The development of clinical guidelines to be used at hospital level is left to clinicians working in the country's main hospital (Mater Dei Hospital). Clinical guidelines in primary care have been developed through a collaboration between a lead practitioner in Family Medicine and relevant specialists from Mater Dei Hospital.	Clinical guidelines development is decentralized. The Department of Medicine at the central hospital developed its own committee (CGCC) to regulate clinical guidelines development. SIGN guidance is also used. Clinical guidelines in primary care have been developed by adapting international clinical guidelines. There is no formal procedure for updating clinical guidelines.

[c] Department of Health Promotion and Disease Prevention, 2010.

Quality control	Enforcement	Implementation	Evaluation
eview processes exist for inical guidelines developed t secondary and primary are levels; however, no pecific instruments are sed to validate them. linical guidelines developed y hospital clinicians ndergo an internal review rocess. or clinical guidelines eveloped in primary care, draft version is circulated mong stakeholders for eedback and amendments.	The use of clinical guidelines is not mandatory. Clinical guidelines used in primary care have to be authorized by the Director of Primary Health.	No formal processes are in place for implementation of clinical guidelines. Clinical guidelines in use at Mater Dei Hospital are available electronically through the hospital intranet.	There is no formal evaluation of clinical guidelines. In hospital they are periodically evaluated by the CGCC.

Country	Definition and regulatory basis	Types and levels	Actors involved	Development process
Netherlands	There is no official basis for the development and implementation of clinical guidelines. Clinical guidelines are produced by different institutions such as the Dutch Council for Quality of Care should work on the harmonization of clinical guidelines development. In 1997 a national platform (EBRO) was initiated by the Dutch Cochrane Centre and the CBO to support the clinical guideline development process and the use of clinical guidelines.	Clinical guideline production is centralized. Additionally, in primary care, the NHG takes a central role in the development of clinical guidelines.	Organizations that produce clinical guidelines are: the RIVM, the CBO, the Dutch Council for Quality of Care, the NHG, Dutch Association of Comprehensive Cancer Centres, the Netherlands Institute of Mental Health & Addiction (Trimbos), the KNGF, and the LEVV. Clinical guidelines are also introduced indirectly by the development and implementation of Disease Management Programmes.	The Dutch Council for Quality of Care conducts the development, implementation and update of guidelines and works on the harmonization of clinical guidelines development. There is no national guidance on methodology to develop clinical guidelines.

Quality control	Enforcement	Implementation	Evaluation
There is no formal methodology for quality assessment. Methods used differ among organizations.	Clinical guidelines use is mandatory only in certain cases, e.g. in end-of-life care.	Some insurers provide financial incentives to support clinical guidelines implementation. Indirectly, legislation on quality of health care organizations or patient–doctor interactions influences the utilization of clinical guidelines on behalf of practitioners. Most organizations have published clinical guidelines on their web sites.	There is no official regulation for the evaluation of clinical guidelines.

Country	Definition and regulatory basis	Types and levels	Actors involved	Development process
Norway	An official basis exists for clinical guideline development and implementation (the Norwegian Directorate of Health). The Directorate is the only institution with a mandate to develop national clinical guidelines.	Clinical guidelines exist on both prevention and treatment of chronic diseases. Official national clinical guidelines are usually developed centrally. The Directorate of Health is responsible for the development of "priority guidelines" in cooperation with Norway's four Regional Health Authorities.	The Norwegian Directorate of Health often works in close cooperation with representatives from relevant specialist groups and other key stakeholders, such as the Norwegian Medicines Agency and patient interest groups. Other guidelines are often developed by the Medical Societies of the Norwegian Medical Association.	The Norwegian Board of Health Supervision has developed a "Guideline for developing clinical guideline" in cooperation with the Norwegian Medical Association and others. The Directorate has also compiled a "Reference book on developing Clinical Guidelines" in cooperation with the Norwegian Electronic Health Library and the Norwegian Knowledge Centre for Health Services. The AGREE instrument is used during the development process. The need for a revision of a national clinical guideline is expected to be considered within three years after the publication of the guideline.

Quality control	Enforcement	Implementation	Evaluation
Clinical guidelines are checked for quality using the AGREE instrument by the Secretariat of the Directorate of Health (Requirement) and the Norwegian Electronic Health Library. Then, clinical guidelines are published online.	The use of national guidelines is not mandatory. The "priority guidelines" also are not considered as binding documents for health service providers. No financial incentives exist for the use of clinical guidelines.	No financial incentives exist for the implementation of national clinical guidelines. The use of clinical guidelines is promoted through web sites, some developed with interactive learning. Certain guidelines related to practical clinical implementation are integrated as IT applications in electronic patient record systems.	No data exist on formal evaluation of clinical guidelines use.

Country	Definition and regulatory basis	Types and levels	Actors involved	Development process
Poland	No national standard or legal basis for clinical guidelines development exists.	The National Pharmaceutical Policy in 2003 identified a need for the development of ambulatory health care formularies, which would contain treatment guidelines. Work on these formularies is still in progress. Clinical guidelines exist for both chronic (e.g. COPD, asthma, hypertension, diabetes) and acute conditions (e.g. pulmonary embolism, DVT).	The development of clinical guidelines is decentralized. Different institutions can be involved in clinical guidelines development: professional organizations, specialists' medical societies, and the CoPFiP.	The clinical guideline development process is not coordinated and guidance on standardizing clinical guidelines development does not exist.
Portugal	A legal basis for clinical guidelines exists. The DGS (a government body) is legally responsible for producing and implementing guidelines. Other decentralized organizations are also involved in developing clinical guidelines. Clinical guidelines are developed and implemented within the framework of government documents, NSFs, within Disease Management Programmes as well as through guidance produced by quasi-official agencies.	Clinical guidelines exist on preventing and treating chronic diseases, as well as for other conditions.	Clinical guidelines development is mostly centralized (through the DGS). The DGS mostly develops clinical guidelines. In addition, several medical societies for sub-specialties and the APMGF also develop clinical guidelines. An attempt to create a body of advisers, including primary care physicians, has recently been initiated.	The DGS often consults with experts, mostly medical specialists. No official guidelines exist for the development process of clinical guidelines, although some academic centres have published best practice recommendations regarding clinical guideline methodology.

Quality control	Enforcement	Implementation	Evaluation
There is no formal methodology for quality assessment and there is no requirement to carry out quality control. The CoPFiP uses the Delphi approach for consensus among the panel of experts and practitioners involved. Some clinical guidelines already include quality checks, e.g. the clinical guidelines for DVT or pulmonary embolism.	The use of clinical guidelines is not mandatory and there are no financial incentives for using them.	No incentives exist to implement clinical guidelines. The CoPFiP has been promoting clinical guidelines use by general practitioners through workshops, seminars, lectures and publications.	The evaluation of clinical guidelines is not mandatory and is only performed to a limited extent. The CoPFiP partially monitors clinical guidelines implementation. Sporadic research projects on the utilization of clinical guidelines have been initiated.
Formal requirements exist for clinical guidelines quality control before implementation.	The use of clinical guidelines is mandatory. Financial incentives exist for doctors, nurses and staff, based on their score in the annual audit of family physician performance (obligatory for family physicians under the new regulations).	The implementation of clinical guidelines is promoted through different disease-specific IT tools (in place for diabetes, child care, hypertension, cancer screening, maternal care and family planning), web sites (e.g. the DGS web site)[b] and accompanying specialist literature.	Evidence on the evaluation of the development, implementation and use of clinical guidelines is available. The performance indicators used in the annual audit of family physician performance are under review by the government.

DGS, 2012.

Country	Definition and regulatory basis	Types and levels	Actors involved	Development process
Romania	The process of clinical guideline production is still in its infancy. The development of clinical guidelines is the responsibility of the Ministry of Health. The actual task is delegated to expert groups from different clinical specialties, officially appointed by the Ministry to provide advice and guidance in their respective fields.	Clinical guidelines exist in general and for chronic conditions in particular, such as for type 2 diabetes mellitus, low lumbar pain, depressive disorders, asthma and malignancies.	The Ministry of Health appointed 10 special commissions comprising medical experts in different medical fields, to develop recommendations in their specialties. Clinical guidelines are also developed by the National Centre for Family Medicine, aimed at family doctors.	No explicit methodology is indicated for the development of clinical guidelines. Commissions have used specifications provided in Ministerial Orders and existing international guidance to form recommendations. Special attention is to be paid to consensus processes. The National Centre for Family Medicine produced a methodology for developing clinical guidelines for its own guidance, involving an evidence-based medicine approach.
Slovakia	No official basis for clinical guidelines development currently exists. In 2004 the NIKI was established, aiming to develop and implement national clinical guidelines. However, clinical guidelines development is not coordinated.	Only a few clinical guidelines exist and usually they consist of translated European recommend-ations. Slovak physicians often refer to guidance produced by the Czech National College of General Practice when national recommend-ations are not at hand.	Clinical guidelines development is both centralized and decentralized. Specialist medical associations (e.g. for cardiology) are clinical guidelines developers. Another clinical guidelines developer is the Central Commission of Rational Pharmacotherapy and Drug Policy of the Ministry of Health. However, their clinical guidelines do not cover the most important chronic conditions.	NIKI published a handbook for developing national clinical guidelines in 2005 (NIKI, 2005a). No further publication has followed the first. It is not mandatory to use the handbook and it is unclear to what extent it is used.

Quality control	Enforcement	Implementation	Evaluation
There is no evidence of clinical guidelines quality control being carried out. However, for the 10 practice guidelines produced by the special commissions, the AGREE instrument was applied before finalization of the guideline to ensure due process had been followed.	Clinicians are expected to implement the clinical guidelines developed by the Ministry of Health. Clinical guidelines produced by the National Centre for Family Medicine are not connected to governmental mandates. Financial incentives operate by means of provider contracts with the Insurance Fund. Health units that have developed and implement treatment protocols based on national guidelines receive additional funding.	No regulated process of implementation exists. Clinical guidelines are available online but there are no other IT tools to facilitate their utilization. Press conferences and publications are used to disseminate clinical guidelines.	There is no indication of evaluation taking place after the publication of a clinical guideline.
No clinical guidelines quality control is carried out.	Guidance utilization is not mandatory but the issue is on the Ministry of Health agenda.	A regulated process of implementation does not exist.	There is no indication of evaluation after clinical guidelines are published.

Country	Definition and regulatory basis	Types and levels	Actors involved	Development process
Slovenia	There is no legal framework or official basis for clinical guidelines development or implementation and no national body is responsible for the clinical guidelines. A proposal that was developed in 2010 to put the Agency for Quality and Safety in charge of clinical guidelines has been abandoned. A new proposal is currently being prepared.	Clinical guidelines are poorly developed and implemented. Often international clinical guidelines are used. A range of recommendations are published in national journals but the methodology behind their development is rarely explained. For other chronic diseases (COPD/asthma), only recommendations/expert opinions on treatment exist.	Clinical guidelines are mainly developed by medical associations for various specialties.	In 2003 the Ministry of Health published the *Manual on development of clinical practice guidelines*[a] which takes into account some methods for clinical guidelines development (SIGN, ÄZQ and G-I-N). However, the manual is often not applied in developing the guidelines. Only a few clinical guidelines (i.e. those for diabetes) explicitly state the level of evidence used. Clinical guidelines are mainly developed based upon the consensus of the experts in a certain field.

[a] Slovenian Ministry of Health, 2003.

Quality control	Enforcement	Implementation	Evaluation
According to the *Manual on development of clinical practice guidelines*, the AGREE tool should be used for quality control. However, as the manual is not often used, currently there is no quality control of clinical guidelines.	Existing guidelines are not mandatory and there are no financial incentives for implementation.	Clinical guidelines are poorly implemented and their implementation is inadequately assessed. Currently, there is no discussion on how to continue with the implementation of clinical guidelines.	There is no quality control and no evaluation of clinical guidelines takes place.

Country	Definition and regulatory basis	Types and levels	Actors involved	Development process
Spain	A specific programme on clinical guidelines has been in place since 2006. The Quality Agency of the Ministry of Health develops a Quality Plan that comprises the strategy of "Improving clinical excellence" and specific objectives related to clinical guidelines.	Clinical guidelines exist on both treatment and prevention. There is a Clinical Practice Guideline Programme in the Spanish National Health System, coordinated by GuíaSalud. In some Autonomous Communities (regions), HTA agencies and units also publish clinical guidelines.	The responsible body for coordinating the development of clinical guidelines is the Ministry of Health and different HTA agencies/ units (within the regions) participate in the process, coordinated by GuíaSalud. The group of agents involved in the development of clinical guidelines includes the following profiles: clinical leaders; other clinical experts such as nurses or pharmacists; experts in the development of clinical practice guidelines; patients'/carers' associations; technical coordinators; and other experts (epidemiologists, health economists, lawyers, qualitative techniques, experts on statistics, etc.). Patient involvement is becoming more common.	The Quality Agency of the Ministry of Health coordinates the development of clinical guidelines through GuíaSalud, establishing agreements with the different HTA agencies/units (within the regions). They are funded through an agreement with the National Quality Agency and each of the agencies responsible for drawing up the clinical guidelines. Methodological experts (experts in the development of clinical guidelines) are usually responsible for systematic reviews, although it depends on each working group. Methodological handbooks (development, updating and implementation) are followed within the Clinical Practice Guideline Programme.

Quality control	Enforcement	Implementation	Evaluation
No mandatory quality control process exists. However, quality control is commonly carried out using the AGREE instrument, together with external reviews. It is a requirement for being included as part of Spanish Guidelines Clearinghouse in the Spanish National Health System, coordinated by GuíaSalud. GuíaSalud has its own criteria to be met before including a clinical guideline in its clearinghouse, but these criteria mostly have their basis in the AGREE instrument.	The use of clinical guidelines is not mandatory within the Autonomous Communities.	There is variability in clinical guidelines implementation. No incentives exist for national-level implementation, although they may exist in some Autonomous Communities. There is also an implementation handbook within the Clinical Practice Guideline Programme. Professional training programmes also address the issue of improving the quality of the clinical guidelines.	No formal control system is in place ensuring the implementation and use of clinical guidelines.

Country	Definition and regulatory basis	Types and levels	Actors involved	Development process
Sweden	The NBHW (an agency under the Ministry of Health and Social Affairs) is responsible for clinical guidelines. However, counties and municipalities also develop clinical guidelines.	Clinical guidelines exist both for chronic and other diseases (e.g. diabetes, renal failure, coronary heart disease, cataract surgery, stroke, hip fracture and hip replacement, and malignant neoplasms). National clinical guidelines exist, along with regional and local guidelines (often based on national guidelines).	Clinical guidelines are developed by the NBHW, counties and municipalities. In addition, the SALAR as well as the SBU is integrated in the development process. Experts in systematic reviews, and economic evaluation, along with a variety of health professionals are involved in the process.	The NBHW selects guidelines to be developed (based on burden of disease, costs and demand from professionals) and provides guidance on development. Then, a pool of experts called a Fact Group is established. This group performs a systematic review of the evidence, while a pool of health economic experts performs a CEA of the intervention. Then, a prioritizing group (consisting of experts on health and medical care) rank the intervention according to the severity of the condition(s) and the evidence produced. The clinical guideline also includes recommendations on measures that should not be implemented at all ("Do Not Do"), in cases in which those particular measures have no effect or may entail risks for the patient.

Quality control	Enforcement	Implementation	Evaluation
A quality assessment is performed but it is not clear which instrument is used.	The use of guidelines is endorsed but no penalties are in place for non-compliance. In some areas, financial incentives are in place.	Several tools exist to facilitate clinical guidelines implementation. The final version of the clinical guidelines is published on the NBHW web site. A short version is compiled for the lay public. Publications, educational materials, conferences, IT applications, or even organizational interventions support the implementation. Moreover, updated clinical guidelines are sent to each registered practitioner.	The final version of a clinical guideline should also include indicators of a good standard of care that can be used to track the improvement in health care after the guidelines' implementation, as well as their impact. The use of clinical guidelines should be regularly evaluated by the NBHW as well as by county councils or universities on request.

Country	Definition and regulatory basis	Types and levels	Actors involved	Development process
Switzerland	There is an official basis for the development of clinical guidelines but no agencies are formally mandated with the development of clinical guidelines. There is no recent evaluation of the number, origin or quality of produced clinical guidelines.	Recommendations for best practice exist on the prevention and treatment of a range of chronic conditions. Most of the clinical guidelines are developed by professional organizations or are adapted versions of international standards by a group of experts. Several local and small initiatives are in place in several cantons.	National societies and associations or small groups of physicians are behind most of the existing best practice recommendations and both institutional and financial support for the development of decision-making aids is limited.	No general guidelines exist for clinical guidelines development. No data are available on the extent to which guideline production, adaptation or implementation are based on best evidence.

Quality control	Enforcement	Implementation	Evaluation
There is no formal quality control of clinical guidelines. The AGREE and ADAPTE instruments are in use by certain hubs, such as the one at the University of Lausanne.	The use of clinical guidelines is not mandatory. No financial incentives exist to encourage the use of clinical guidelines.	There is no nationwide implementation of clinical guidelines. Some local directives on medical services in certain hospitals exist. No centrally or widely distributed tools exist to assist professionals and patients in their decision making. Most related initiatives exist on a local basis and their dissemination is therefore limited.	No control system is in place ensuring the implementation and use of clinical guidelines.

Country	Definition and regulatory basis	Types and levels	Actors involved	Development process
United Kingdom (England)	There is an official basis for the development of clinical guidelines. The Department of Health established the NICE in 1999 to develop clinical guidelines. The Institute subsequently developed a comprehensive manual for clinical guideline development.	Clinical guidelines exist for several conditions, both chronic and not, for both management and prevention.	All clinical guidelines are developed by the NICE in consultation with independent committees and experts working in health care, academia and industry, alongside patients and members of the public with a background or interest in the area. The NCCCC, funded by the NICE, leads on developing clinical guidelines for the treatment of chronic conditions. The Centre for Public Health Excellence provides guidance on services that contribute to the prevention of chronic conditions and encourage good health and well-being. Members of the GDG are required to undergo formal training on the guideline development process.	Clinical guideline topics are referred by the Department of Health and health care professionals. The guideline development process is based on the AGREE instrument and is evidence based. The NCC commissioned for the clinical guidelines prepares the scope. An independent GDG is established: members are recruited through formal adverts on the NICE web site. Conflict of interest must be declared by members throughout the whole process. The GDG critically appraises the evidence. The NICE experts carry out a statistical and health economics review. The draft goes through at least one public consultation period. An independent guideline review panel validates the clinical guideline. Guidelines are normally considered for an update three years after publication but partial updates may be carried out earlier than this if significant new evidence emerges.

Quality control	Enforcement	Implementation	Evaluation
Quality control is performed using the AGREE instrument. The stakeholder consultation, expert reviews and assessment by the independent guideline review panel are all part of the validation process. Prior to publication, the guidelines are subjected to an internal quality control assessment at the Centre for Clinical Practice. NHS Evidence Quality also assesses guidance. The NICE Guidance Executive approves the final version of the guideline before it goes for publication.	Clinical guidelines are not mandatory. However, health care professionals are expected to take NICE clinical guidelines fully into account when exercising their clinical judgement and they are expected to record their reasons for not following clinical guideline recommendations. All NHS organizations are expected to meet NICE standards to ensure that everyone receives the same quality of care.	Clinical guidelines may be adapted and implemented at the local level through NHS Hospital Trusts, PCTs, local authorities and voluntary organizations. The NICE supports the implementation of clinical guidelines and it has a team of implementation consultants that work nationally to share learning and to support education and training. There is a range of implementation tools available through the NICE web site, where practitioners share their innovative and successful approaches to implementing clinical guidelines.	The NICE produces implementation reports which measure the uptake of specific recommendations. Interested researchers assess the uptake and effectiveness of guidance on an adhoc basis. Reports are collated by the NICE in a central searchable database.

Case studies on the development of clinical guidelines for type 2 diabetes mellitus – template for data collection

BACKGROUND INFORMATION

a) Do clinical guidelines on preventing and/or treating TD2M exist in your country (possibly under another name)?
b) If not: (i) Do they exist for other types of diseases or interventions?
c) (ii) Are there any other tools to assist professionals and patients in making appropriate decisions for patients with TD2M?
d) Is there a database of existing guidelines on diabetes?
e) Are different aspects of the management of TD2M presented in separate guidelines (for instance, diabetes footcare)?
f) If that is the case, how is this coordinated?

REGULATORY BASIS

a) Is there an official basis for the development and implementation of TD2M guidelines in your country (e.g. legal basis, government document or statement by an ALB or quasi-official agency – possibly the same as for HTA)?
b) If yes, which?
c) If no, are there any proposals to create such a basis?

FOR THE DEVELOPMENT OF CLINICAL GUIDELINES FOR TD2M

a) Are TD2M guidelines developed centrally, or is the process decentralized? Is this process representative of guideline development in general in your country?
b) If it is carried out centrally, by whom?
c) If the process is decentralized, who develops TD2M clinical guidelines (e.g. professional organizations or individual groups of physicians)? Is the decentralized process coordinated (e.g. by an association of professional bodies or an ALB)?
d) Are there guidelines for TD2M clinical guideline development and if so who provides those? Is that also the case for clinical guidelines in general?
e) What disciplines does the GDG include (librarians, epidemiologists, health economists, statisticians, etc.)?
f) Which types of clinicians (from which specialties) are involved in the development of clinical guidelines for TD2M?
g) How is the clinical guideline development funded?

FOR THE DEVELOPMENT OF CLINICAL GUIDELINES FOR TD2M (contd)

h) Who undertakes systematic reviews and critical appraisal of evidence?
i) Does the GDG undergo methodological training?
j) Are patients involved or consulted in guideline development (e.g. participation in the GDG, surveys of patient views/preferences, review by representatives of patients' organizations)?
k) How is consensus achieved?
l) Is there a procedure for updating guidelines? If so, how often do updates take place?
m) Does your country participate in any international collaboration for guideline development?
n) Are guidelines from other countries used? If so, are these reviewed/re-edited or tested for applicability in the new context?

ALL THESE QUESTIONS FOR CLINICAL GUIDELINES ON TYPE 2 DIABETES MELLITUS

QUALITY CONTROL

a) Are clinical guidelines checked for quality before being implemented (e.g. using the AGREE instrument)?
b) If so, who performs the task (i.e. the same body that developed the clinical guidelines, or a separate entity)?
c) Is quality control a requirement for implementation and, if so, by whom?
d) Are guidelines piloted or tested against agreed quality criteria before being adopted for implementation? What is the final process of guideline authorization?

IMPLEMENTATION

a) Is the use of (certain) guidelines mandatory?
b) If yes, who regulates that?
c) If not, are there incentives to implement and use clinical guidelines (e.g. financial, through contracts between purchasers and providers)?
d) Are there IT applications or other tools to promote clinical guideline application (e.g. E3e)?
e) At what level do clinical guidelines usually operate (e.g. local, national, EU/ international)?
f) What is the process by which a health care professional will be able to use a clinical guideline?
g) Is there a programme to help support implementation of clinical guidelines (e.g. to ensure dissemination to target audiences, actively engage with stakeholders and users of guidelines, share learning and educational material)?
h) Are clinical guidelines being used in conjunction with other tools to assist practitioner and patient decisions about appropriate health care for specific circumstances?
i) Are there any complementary tools developed in conjunction with clinical guidelines to support their implementation (e.g. clinical/care pathways)?

EVALUATION

a) Are the development, quality control, implementation and use of clinical guidelines evaluated?
b) If yes by whom and how often?
c) If yes, what criteria is the evaluation based on?
d) Is it a requirement and, if so, by whom?
e) Is the use and/or impact of clinical guidelines monitored and/or evaluated? Are there any studies and/or reports on such evaluations (e.g. data on use of guidelines, impact on health outcome, teamwork, patient/provider satisfaction)?
f) Are there any reports on the key contextual factors (e.g. organizational culture, acceptance by the medical/health care professions) or other factors that might support or hinder the implementation of guidelines in your country?
g) What changes have there been in the development, implementation and use of guidelines in the last 10 years? Are there plans for further developments related to clinical guidelines in your country?

Annex 3

Systematic review methods tables

Table A3.1 *Search strategy*

Chronic conditions (searched in Text, Abstract, Keyword)	Coronary heart diseases [MeSH term] OR Cardiovascular diseases [MeSH term]
	Diabetes
	Asthma
	COPD
	Breast cancer [MeSH term]
	Cervical cancer [MeSH term]
	Colorectal carcinoma [MeSH term]
	Depressive disorder
Countries (searched in Text, Abstract, Keyword, Country of publication, Address of author)	Austria, Belgium, Bulgaria, Cyprus, Czech Republic, Denmark, Estonia, Finland, France, Germany, Greece, Hungary, Ireland, Italy, Latvia, Lithuania, Luxembourg, Malta, Netherlands, Poland, Portugal, Romania, Slovakia, Slovenia, Spain, Sweden, United Kingdom, EU, Europe
Topic (searched in Text, Abstract, Keyword)	Guideline OR clinical guideline
Year of publication	From 2000 to 2011

Table A3.2 *Data extracted from the studies*

Study ID

Aim

European countries implemented or included in the analysis

Health conditions

Guidelines information

Year of study implementation

Setting

Study design

Study duration

Table A3.2 *contd*

For guidelines evaluation studies
Number of guidelines
Clinical domain
Guideline for which level of care
Outcome
Discussion

For implementations/Impact studies
Participants (number)
Number of interventions
Description of the intervention
Intervention Group 1 (number, description)
Intervention Group 2 (number, description)
Control Group (number, description)
Outcome (primary and secondary)
Outcome assessment
Results: quantitative data
Barriers to implementation
Discussion: author note

Table A3.3 *EMBASE search results*

	Searches	Results
2	(Coronary Heart Diseases or Cardiovascular Diseases or Coronary Diseases or Diabetes or Asthma or COPD or Chronic Obstructive Pulmonary Disease or Arthritis or Breast Neoplasm or Breast Tumour or Mammary Carcinoma or Breast Cancer or Cervical Neoplasm or Cervix Neoplasm or Cancer of the Uterine Cervix or Cancer of the Cervix or Cervical Cancer or Cervix Cancer or Colorectal Tumour or Colorectal Neoplasm or Colorectal Carcinoma or Colorectal Cancer or Chronic Lymphocytic Leukaemia or Depressive disorder).ab. or (Coronary Heart Diseases or Cardiovascular Diseases or Coronary Diseases or Diabetes or Asthma or COPD or Chronic Obstructive Pulmonary Disease or Arthritis or Breast Neoplasm or Breast Tumour or Mammary Carcinoma or Breast Cancer or Cervical Neoplasm or Cervix Neoplasm or Cancer of the Uterine Cervix or Cancer of the Cervix or Cervical Cancer or Cervix Cancer or Colorectal Tumour or Colorectal Neoplasm or Colorectal Carcinoma or Colorectal Cancer or Chronic Lymphocytic Leukaemia or Depressive disorder).ti. or (Coronary Heart Diseases or Cardiovascular Diseases or Coronary Diseases or Diabetes or Asthma or COPD or Chronic Obstructive Pulmonary Disease or Arthritis or Breast Neoplasm or Breast Tumour or Mammary Carcinoma or Breast Cancer or Cervical Neoplasm or Cervix Neoplasm or Cancer of the Uterine Cervix or Cancer of the Cervix or Cervical Cancer or Cervix Cancer or Colorectal Tumour or Colorectal Neoplasm or Colorectal Carcinoma or Colorectal Cancer or Chronic Lymphocytic Leukaemia or Depressive disorder).kw.	931 244

Table A3.3 *contd*

Searches	Results
3 (Austria or Belgium or Bulgaria or Cyprus or Czech Republic or Denmark or Estonia or Finland or France or Germany or Greece or Hungary or Ireland or Italy or Latvia or Lithuania or Luxembourg or Malta or Netherlands or Poland or Portugal or Romania or Slovakia or Slovenia or Spain or Sweden or United Kingdom or EU or Europe).ab. or (Austria or Belgium or Bulgaria or Cyprus or Czech Republic or Denmark or Estonia or Finland or France or Germany or Greece or Hungary or Ireland or Italy or Latvia or Lithuania or Luxembourg or Malta or Netherlands or Poland or Portugal or Romania or Slovakia or Slovenia or Spain or Sweden or United Kingdom or EU or Europe).ti. or (Austria or Belgium or Bulgaria or Cyprus or Czech Republic or Denmark or Estonia or Finland or France or Germany or Greece or Hungary or Ireland or Italy or Latvia or Lithuania or Luxembourg or Malta or Netherlands or Poland or Portugal or Romania or Slovakia or Slovenia or Spain or Sweden or United Kingdom or EU or Europe).kw. or (Austria or Belgium or Bulgaria or Cyprus or Czech Republic or Denmark or Estonia or Finland or France or Germany or Greece or Hungary or Ireland or Italy or Latvia or Lithuania or Luxembourg or Malta or Netherlands or Poland or Portugal or Romania or Slovakia or Slovenia or Spain or Sweden or United Kingdom or EU or Europe).cp. or (Austria or Belgium or Bulgaria or Cyprus or Czech Republic or Denmark or Estonia or Finland or France or Germany or Greece or Hungary or Ireland or Italy or Latvia or Lithuania or Luxembourg or Malta or Netherlands or Poland or Portugal or Romania or Slovakia or Slovenia or Spain or Sweden or United Kingdom or EU or Europe).ad.	11 252 745
4 (Guideline or clinical guideline).ab. or (Guideline or clinical guideline).ti. or (Guideline or clinical guideline).kw.	24 611
5 2 and 3 and 4	1 389
6 limit 5 to (yr="2000–2011" and (adult <18 to 64 years> or aged <65+ years>))	352

Table A3.4 *MEDLINE search results*

Searches	Results
2 (Coronary Heart Diseases or Cardiovascular Diseases or Coronary Diseases or Diabetes or Asthma or COPD or Chronic Obstructive Pulmonary Disease or Arthritis or Breast Neoplasm or Breast Tumour or Mammary Carcinoma or Breast Cancer or Cervical Neoplasm or Cervix Neoplasm or Cancer of the Uterine Cervix or Cancer of the Cervix or Cervical Cancer or Cervix Cancer or Colorectal Tumour or Colorectal Neoplasm or Colorectal Carcinoma or Colorectal Cancer or Chronic Lymphocytic Leukaemia or Depressive disorder).ab. or (Coronary Heart Diseases or Cardiovascular Diseases or Coronary Diseases or Diabetes or Asthma or COPD or Chronic Obstructive Pulmonary Disease or Arthritis or Breast Neoplasm or Breast Tumour or Mammary Carcinoma or Breast Cancer or Cervical Neoplasm or Cervix Neoplasm or Cancer of the Uterine Cervix or Cancer of the Cervix or Cervical Cancer or Cervix Cancer or Colorectal Tumour or Colorectal Neoplasm or Colorectal Carcinoma or Colorectal Cancer or Chronic Lymphocytic Leukaemia or Depressive disorder).kw. or (Coronary Heart Diseases or Cardiovascular Diseases or Coronary Diseases or Diabetes or Asthma or COPD or Chronic Obstructive Pulmonary Disease or Arthritis or Breast Neoplasm or Breast Tumour or Mammary Carcinoma or Breast Cancer or Cervical Neoplasm or Cervix Neoplasm or Cancer of the Uterine Cervix or Cancer of the Cervix or Cervical Cancer or Cervix Cancer or Colorectal Tumour or Colorectal Neoplasm or Colorectal Carcinoma or Colorectal Cancer or Chronic Lymphocytic Leukaemia or Depressive disorder).ti.	720 513
4 (Austria or Belgium or Bulgaria or Cyprus or Czech Republic or Denmark or Estonia or Finland or France or Germany or Greece or Hungary or Ireland or Italy or Latvia or Lithuania or Luxembourg or Malta or Netherlands or Poland or Portugal or Romania or Slovakia or Slovenia or Spain or Sweden or United Kingdom or EU or Europe).ab. or (Austria or Belgium or Bulgaria or Cyprus or Czech Republic or Denmark or Estonia or Finland or France or Germany or Greece or Hungary or Ireland or Italy or Latvia or Lithuania or Luxembourg or Malta or Netherlands or Poland or Portugal or Romania or Slovakia or Slovenia or Spain or Sweden or United Kingdom or EU or Europe).kw. or (Austria or Belgium or Bulgaria or Cyprus or Czech Republic or Denmark or Estonia or Finland or France or Germany or Greece or Hungary or Ireland or Italy or Latvia or Lithuania or Luxembourg or Malta or Netherlands or Poland or Portugal or Romania or Slovakia or Slovenia or Spain or Sweden or United Kingdom or EU or Europe).ti. or (Austria or Belgium or Bulgaria or Cyprus or Czech Republic or Denmark or Estonia or Finland or France or Germany or Greece or Hungary or Ireland or Italy or Latvia or Lithuania or Luxembourg or Malta or Netherlands or Poland or Portugal or Romania or Slovakia or Slovenia or Spain or Sweden or United Kingdom or EU or Europe).cp.	3 833 292
5 (Guideline or clinical guideline).ab. or (Guideline or clinical guideline).kw. or (Guideline or clinical guideline).ti.	18 586
6 2 and 4 and 5	555
7 limit 6 to yr="2000–Current"	523
8 limit 7 to humans	491
10 (Journal article not Review).pt.	17 640 096
11 8 and 10	398

Table A3.5 *Excluded studies and reason for exclusion from work relating to the implementation of clinical guidelines*

Implementation: excluded studies	Reason for exclusion
Bell et al., 2000 Hermens, Hak & Hulscher, 2001	Study design
Bouaud et al., 2001 Kuilboer et al., 2006	Use of computer system
Dijkstra et al., 2006	CEA
Lundborg et al., 2000	Self-reported data
Martens et al., 2006 Martens et al., 2007	Comparison of devices, not guidelines
Meulepas et al., 2007	Participants: not physicians
Sinnema et al., 2011	Protocol of an ongoing study
Witt et al., 2004	Age group: children

Table A3.6 *Excluded studies and reason for exclusion from work relating to the health impact of clinical guidelines*

Impact: excluded studies	Reason for exclusion
Gitt et al., 2011	Adherence at hospital level
Varga et al., 2010 Wockel et al., 2010	Breast cancer treatment at hospital
Schaapveld et al., 2005	Breast cancer treatment according to node biopsy result
Cobos et al., 2005	Only data on CEA
Lagerlov et al., 2000a Wiener-Ogilvie et al., 2007	Qualitative data (knowledge)
Karbach et al., 2011	Qualitative data (knowledge) and survey on adherence
Manchon-Walsh et al., 2011	Rectal cancer treatment at hospital
Aakre et al., 2010 De Marco et al., 2005 Federici et al., 2006 Glaab et al., 2006a Glaab et al., 2006b Kamposioras et al., 2008 Pont et al., 2004 Ratsep et al., 2006 Tabrizi, 2009 Wagner et al., 2004 Winnefeld & Bruggeman, 2008	Self-reported outcome
Bakx et al., 2003 Benhamou et al., 2009 Ernst, Kinnear & Hudson, 2005 Ganten & Raspe, 2003 Hartmann et al., 2008 Juul et al., 2009 Kamyar et al., 2008 Peters-Klimm et al., 2008 Sarc et al., 2011 Smolders et al., 2009 Smolders et al., 2010 Toti et al., 2007 Tsagaraki, Markantonis & Amfilochiou, 2006 Van Steenbergen et al., 2009 Waldmann et al., 2007 Zink, Huscher & Schneider, 2010	Survey on adherence data

Table A3.7 *Excluded studies and reason for exclusion from the development section*

Impact: excluded studies	Reason for exclusion
Alonso-Coello et al., 2010 Burgers, Cluzeau et al., 2003 Burgers, Grol et al., 2003b	Systematic review with pooled data
Alonso-Coello et al., 2008 Burls, 2010 Schunemann et al., 2009 Schwarz & Lindstrom, 2011	Editorial
Brouwers et al., 2010a Brouwers et al., 2010b Brouwers et al., 2010c	Description of AGREE II
Burgers et al., 2002 Lindström et al., 2010 Pajunen et al., 2010 Paulweber et al., 2010	It is not an analysis of guidelines
Delgado-Noguera et al., 2009 Devroey et al., 2004 Gaebel et al., 2005 Giorgi et al., 2001 Harpole et al., 2003 Navarro Puerto et al., 2008	Out of scope because of the considered condition
Schwarz et al., 2007	Describes a project protocol
Smith et al., 2003	Does not use AGREE instrument
Vergnenegre, 2003	Guide on how to conduct AGREE analysis
Vlayen et al., 2005	Relates to appraisal instruments themselves
Voellinger et al., 2003	Results do not included desired outcomes

Table A3.8 *Characteristics of included studies for evaluating the effectiveness of implementation strategies*

ID	Country Study design Year	Conditions	Guidelines	Participants
Asmar, 2007	France RCT 2004–2005	Hypertension	European Society of Hypertension – International Society of Hypertension guidelines (2003)	Intervention: 502 physicians, 2 128 patients Control: 595 physicians, 2 308 patients
Baker et al., 2003	United Kingdom c-RCT 1998–1999	Asthma and. Stable angina	North of England Guideline Development Project (1996)	Full version: 27 general practitioners Asthma: 896 patients pre, 958 post Angina: 780 patients pre, 787 post Review criteria: 27 general practitioners Asthma: 889 patients pre, 950 post Angina: 792 patients pre, 818 post Review criteria plus feedback: 27 general practitioners Asthma: 894 patients pre, 914 post Angina: 818 patients pre, 807 post
Frijling et al., 2002	Netherlands c-RCT 1996–1998	Type 2 diabetes mellitus	NHG's guidelines on type 2 diabetes mellitus (1989)	124 practices, 185 general practitioners
Hormigo Pozo et al., 2009	Spain CBA 2005	Type 2 diabetes mellitus	Expert's team + European guidelines on hypertension + JNC VII + NCEP + CEIPC + EBM + ESCARDIO Recommendation on anti-platelet treatment (2002–2004)	2 health centres Patients: Intervention 117 Control 118

Multifaceted number intervention	Intervention	Outcome	Effect	Effect sizes[a]
YES 3	Educational outreach visits + Workshops + Educational material for general practitioners	Health impact: • % of patients with blood pressure controlled according to the target level	Significant improvement (Intervention 47.8% versus 44.7% (P– 0.005).	++
YES 2	Feedback + Educational material for general practitioners	Performance criteria: Asthma • Correct asthma diagnosis • Check treatment compliance • Check required dosage • Cheapest formulation of drug used • Check patient's inhaler technique • Record smoking status Angina • Correct diagnosis of angina • Check serum cholesterol • Measure, record and manage blood pressure • Record smoking status • Check patients' drugs compliance • Cheapest formulation of drug used • Correct drug dosage prescribed • Record weight/BMI	No effect	-
YES 3	Educational outreach visits + Feedback + Educational material for general practitioners	Process of care and prescription: • Body weight controlled • Drugs problems discussed • Blood pressure measured • Foot examination • Eye examination • Correct anti-diabetic prescription • Scheduling a follow-up appointment	Significant improvement 2/7 indicators: • Foot examination (1.68, 95% CI 1.19–2.39) • Eye examination (1.52, 95% CI 1.07–2.16)	+
YES 4	Feedback + Workshops + Educational material for general practitioners + Formal training	Process of care and prescription: • % of cardiovascular risk assessment in high-risk population • Medication appropriateness (antihypertensive and anti-platelet)	Significant improvement: • Cardiovascular risk assessment relative risk: 9.74, 95% CI 5.15–18.43 P= 0.0001 • Appropriate anti-platelet treatment relative risk: 1.41, 95% CI 1.04–1,89 P= 0.026	++

Table A3.8 *contd*

ID	Country Study design Year	Conditions	Guidelines	Participants
Lagerlov et al., 2000b	Norway c-RCT 1995	Asthma	Adapted from Guidelines on management of asthma BTS, British Paediatric Association, RCP (1993)	Intervention: 100 general practitioners Control: 99 general practitioners
Perria et al., 2007	Italy c-RCT 2004	Type 2 diabetes mellitus	Adapted from French guidelines: Stratégie de prise en charge du patient diabétique de type 2 à l'exclusion de la prise en charge des complications (2000)	Active implementation: 84 general practitioners, 1 952 patients Passive implementation: 85 general practitioners, 2 106 patients Control: 83 general practitioners, 2 232 patients
Roseman et al., 2007	Germany c-RCT 2005	Osteoarthritis	Adapted from European guidelines (EULAR) 2001	Intervention: 25 general practitioners, 345 patients Control: 25 general practitioners, 332 patients
Sondergaard et al., 2002	Denmark RCT 1998–1999	Asthma	Drug index published by the Danish Medical Association (1998)	Patient count data: 77 general practitioners Aggregated data: 74 general practitioners Control: 141 general practitioners

Multifaceted number intervention	Intervention	Outcome	Effect	Effect sizes[a]
YES 3	Feedback + Workshops + Educational material for general practitioners	Drugs prescriptions: • Medication appropriateness	Significant Improvement: • Relative difference in acceptably treated patients 5.9% (variance 2.5), P= 0.018	+
NO	Training	Process of care and prescription • % of patients with trimester control of HbA1c% • % of patients with macrovascular complications assessment tests (ECG, lipid profile, total cholesterol, HDL cholesterol, tryglicerides) • % of patients with microvascular complications assessment tests (eye examination, serum creatinine, creatinine clearance, microalbuminuria) • % of patients receiving correct drugs according to BMI and age • % of patients with cardiovascular risk receiving correct drugs • % of patients with high blood pressure receiving correct drugs • % of patients with dyslipidemia receiving lipid-lowering drugs	No effect	-
YES 2	Workshops + Educational material for patients	Health impact: quality of life Process of care: • Medication appropriateness • Health care utilization: referrals to orthopaedists, imaging, inpatient care, physiotherapy • Physical activity	Health impact: No difference Process of care: improvement in two processes of care (no. of radiographs and % of prescriptions (P= 0.001))	+
NO	Feedback	Drugs prescriptions: • Medication appropriateness	No effect	-

Table A3.8 *contd*

ID	Country Study design Year	Conditions	Guidelines	Participants
Van Bruggen et al., 2008	Netherlands c-RCT not stated	Type 2 diabetes mellitus	Locally adapted from the Practice guideline type 2 diabetes mellitus of the NHG (1999)	Intervention: 15 general practitioner practices, 822 patients Control: 15 general practitioner practices, 818 patients
Verstappen et al., 2003	Netherlands c-RCT 1999	Cardiovascular/ Hypertension or COPD/ asthma + degenerative joint complaints	National guidelines of the NHG	13 practices (each arm) CV/Hypertension: 85 general practitioners COPD/Asthma + degenerative joint disease: 89 general practitioners

Notes: JNC VII: 7th report of the JNC; ᵃ Effect sizes: "++": mostly effective – there was a significant effect on more than 50% of the indicators; "+": partly effective – there was a significant effect on 50% or less of the indicators; "-": not effective, no significant effect was demonstrated for any of the indicators.

Multifaceted number intervention	Intervention	Outcome	Effect	Effect sizes[a]
NO	Educational outreach visits	Health Impact: • % of patients with poor glycaemic control at baseline that achieved control • Mean HbA1c% value • Total cholesterol value • Blood pressure values • Quality of life Process of care: • Trimester measurements of FBG • Blood pressure control • Body weight control • Medication appropriateness in case of microalbuminuria	Health impact: No difference except in cholesterol: small, statistically significant improvement	+
YES 3	Feedback + Workshops + Educational material for general practitioners	Process of care: • Decrease in the total numbers of requested tests per 6 months per physician • Decrease in the numbers of inappropriate tests as defined in the guidelines	Significant result only in the total number of tests dropped for cardiovascular diseases (P= 0.01)	+

Afterword: the Latin American perspective

Contrary to public perception, infectious diseases cause only less than one-quarter of the deaths in Latin America, while noncommunicable diseases are the leading cause of death in the region – they account for 70% of deaths.[15,16] In fact, it is projected that Latin America will experience substantially greater challenges from the growing noncommunicable disease epidemic. By 2015, obesity rates are expected to increase to as high as 39% in all adults,[17] and by 2020, the predominance of noncommunicable diseases over infectious diseases is to become significantly greater.[18] Furthermore, while serious efforts have been made to thwart tobacco consumption in the region, over half of the 120 million smokers in Latin America will die from a tobacco-related disease.[19] Thus, even if tobacco consumption is eliminated in the region today, Latin American countries would still have the burden of addressing the resulting tobacco-related chronic ailments suffered by former smokers.

The gravity of this reality is further exacerbated by the fact that noncommunicable diseases pose a serious threat to the region's economic development.[20] As it is, Latin America has the highest level of social inequity as compared to other regions,[21] and noncommunicable diseases cut across socio-economic lines, where the poor are the most affected as they are the least able to prevent and treat noncommunicable diseases.[22] Likewise, noncommunicable diseases are

15 Pan-American Health Organization (2011). Las enfermedades no transmisibles en la región de las Américas: todos los sectores de la sociedad pueden ayudar a resolver el problema – informe temático sobre enfermedades no transmisibles. (http://new.paho.org/hq/index.php?option=com_docman&task=doc_download&gid=16160&Itemid=270&lang=en, accessed 21 March 2013), 2.

16 Fernando G. De Maio (2011). Understanding chronic noncommunicable diseases in Latin America: towards an equitybased research agenda. *Globalization and Health*, 7:36, 4.

17 GBC Health (2012). NCDs in Latin America & The Caribbean, 1.

18 Perel, P., Casas, J.P.; Ortiz, Z., Miranda, J.J. (2006). Noncommunicable Diseases and Injuries in Latin America and the Caribbean: Time for Action" (2006). *PLoS medicine*, 3(9), 1448.

19 O'Neill Institute for National and Global Health Law (2012). Tobacco Industry Strategy in Latin American Courts: A Litigation Guide" (http://www.law.georgetown.edu/oneillinstitute/documents/2012_OneillTobaccoLitGuide_ENG.PDF, accessed 21 March 2013), 12.

20 Maio, 1.

21 Perel et. al, 1449.

22 Bloomberg School of Public Health Johns Hopkins University (2009). Non-Communicable Chronic Diseases in Latin America and the Caribbean (http://www.healthycaribbean.org/publications/documents/NCD-in-LAC-USAID.pdf, accessed 21 March 2013), 7.

having a major impact on the working-age population – those between 15 and 60 years of age.[23,24] Moreover, health systems are experiencing a rapidly growing "double burden of disease" represented by noncommunicable diseases and infectious diseases.[25]

Therefore, Latin American countries are inevitably faced with having to control the epidemic through both prevention and patient care management measures. Just as the European Union is seeking to effectively respond to the epidemic by first understanding the landscape of practices based on national clinical guidelines and their impact on patient care and outcomes, Latin America as a region can greatly benefit from a similar undertaking, where the model can be adapted to the realities of the region and a unified response to noncommunicable diseases is developed.

Oscar A. Cabrera, Executive Director/Visiting Professor, and Ana S. Ayala,
Institute Associate

O'Neill Institute for National and Global Health Law
Georgetown University Law Center

---

23 Id.

24 Maio, 5.

25 Bloomberg School of Public Health Johns Hopkins University, 11.